ESTROGEN

By Lila Nachtigall with Joan R. Heilman

The Lila Nachtigall Report

By Joan Rattner Heilman

Having a Cesarean Baby
(with Richard Hausknecht, M.D.)

Diabetes: Controlling It the Easy Way
(with Stanley Mirsky, M.D.)

Bluebird Rescue

The Complete University Medical Diet
(with Maria Simonson, Ph.D.)

Ford Models' Crash Course in Looking Great
(with Eileen Ford)

ESTROGEN
THE FACTS CAN CHANGE YOUR LIFE

---

*The latest word on what the new, safe
estrogen therapy can do for*

Great sex

Strong bones

Good looks

Longer life

Preventing hot flashes

LiLA NACHTiGALL, M.d.
ANd
JOAN RATTNER HEILMAN

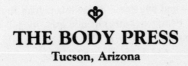

THE BODY PRESS
Tucson, Arizona

Published by The Body Press
A division of HPBooks, Inc.
P.O. Box 5367, Tucson, AZ 85703 (602) 888-2150
©1986 by Lila E. Nachtigall and Joan Rattner Heilman
Designed by Lydia Link
Published by arrangement with Harper & Row, Publishers, Inc.

Library of Congress Cataloging-in-Publication Data

Nachtigall, Lila
  Estrogen: the facts can change your life.

  Reprint. Originally published: New York: Harper & Row, ©1986.
  1. Estrogen—Therapeutic use.   2. Menopause.
3. Women—Healthy and hygiene.   I. Heilman, Joan Rattner.
II. Title [DNLM: 1. Estrogens—therapeutic use—popular works.
2. Menopause—popular works. WP 580 N124e 1986a]
RG186.N28   1986   618.1'75061   87-15859
ISBN 0-89586-630-7 (pbk.)

Printed in United States of America
10 9 8 7 6 5 4 3 2 1

To my children—Margaret, Lisa, and Ellen—and to
my mother, Adele Holzer Ehrenstein

Together they taught me the
joys of motherhood.

CONTENTS

This book is designed to provide general information about estrogen replacement therapy, but it is not intended as a substitute for the advice of your own physician. Because each situation is unique, you should consult your physician to obtain individual information and answers to any questions on symptoms or appropriate medication.

1

Estrogen: Should You or Shouldn't You?

If you're confused about taking estrogen after menopause, wondering if you really need it or whether it's safe, you are certainly not alone. Estrogen replacement confuses most women today. It even confounds most doctors. Can most of the minor discomforts and major health problems of menopause be blamed on lack of estrogen? Is estrogen replacement therapy the *only* way to protect your bones from the ravages of osteoporosis? Is it the *only* way to preserve your sex life? Can it keep your arteries in younger and healthier condition? Does it banish unrelenting vaginal and urinary infections? Will it keep you younger-looking? Is it the best method of eliminating hot flashes, insomnia, strange skin sensations, and the other uncomfortable menopausal symptoms?

Even if the answer to all these questions is *yes*—which it is—even if estrogen does all these wonderful things, is it worth it? Is it safe? Won't it cause cancer or other dire diseases? You recall what you read a few years back about its dangers, and on the other hand, you've heard recently that respected physicians and institutions once more recommend that women take it.

What can you believe? Should you take estrogen or shouldn't you?

In this book, you'll get the absolutely last word, the most up-to-the-minute scientific information available about estrogen replacement therapy (ERT)—what it can and cannot do for you—so you can make an informed decision for yourself. You will find out the trade-offs if you decide against it and all the available alternatives, natural and otherwise, to ERT. And, most important, you'll learn the facts about menopause so you will know what happens to your body when you lose the primary source of your female hormones.

This book will tell you exactly *how* to take estrogen—if you need it and want it—so you needn't worry about your future health. ERT has radically changed in the last decade. It is safe today. In fact, it's *better* than safe. Taking estrogen correctly—combined with progesterone, the second major female hormone—will not increase your chances of uterine cancer and instead will actually help protect you *against* it.

WHO AM I TO TALK?

First, my credentials: I am a physician, a reproductive endocrinologist (a specialist in female hormones), and Associate Professor of Obstetrics and Gynecology at New York University Medical Center, one of the most prestigious and respected medical centers in the world. I am also Director of Gynecologic Endocrinology at New York's Goldwater Memorial Hospital and of Bellevue Hospital Outpatient Services. At Goldwater, I headed the team that made the first long-term prospective study of the effects of estrogen replacement therapy (ERT) on women's health.

As a physician, I see hundreds of menopausal women, as well as younger women with hormone-related problems, every year. As a scientist, I have been involved in the research behind almost every new development in estrogen replacement therapy over the last two decades.

All this doesn't mean I know everything about estrogen, but it means I probably know everything there *is* to know about it at this moment. And I am going to share what I know with you. Because I am under no obligation to any pharmaceutical company and have no financial interest in any product, the information will be as scientifically honest and unbiased as we can possibly make it.

FEAR OF ESTROGEN: IS IT VALID?

Because of my specialty, both physicians and women constantly come to me looking for information about menopause and estrogen. I don't feel my day is complete if I am not asked at least five times for my position on estrogen replacement therapy.

I see women every week who are desperate and miserable because of menopausal symptoms and physical changes so uncomfortable that they can't function normally. But their friends and relatives warn them to stay away from estrogen—"You'll get cancer!"—and even their doctors don't have the answers to their questions about it.

Take Mrs. G., for example. When she first came to me about six months after her menopause, she was having 30 to 40 drenching hot flashes every day and night. She had serious insomnia, never got a good night's sleep. She suffered from alarming palpitations. And because she had menopause early, at 41, and had a small frame, she was a likely candidate for developing osteoporosis, the brittle-bones disease, and for losing her ability to have normal sexual intercourse by the time she reached 55.

But she was terrified of estrogen. "Oh no," she said vehemently, "I wouldn't take that. It gives you cancer."

What she didn't know was that if she took estrogen correctly—as we will explain here—she was *less* likely to get cancer than she was before.

Estrogen replacement therapy is absolutely safe when it is used correctly in the new medically proven way (in low doses, combined with progesterone, prescribed individually, and monitored regularly)—and we are going to tell you why this is so.

Here are the most important facts about estrogen replacement therapy as we know them now:

ERT taken correctly will not give you cancer. Instead, it helps protect you against it. The incidence of both uterine and breast cancer has been found to be significantly *lower* among women on estrogen/progesterone therapy than among those who don't take hormones.

On the average, women on ERT tend to live longer than other women. They suffer fewer heart attacks, and have only a third of the risk of dying from coronary heart disease because estrogen helps keep the artery walls clear of plaque.

Chapter 2 will give you the details.

MORE WOMEN CAN TAKE ESTROGEN NOW

Even women who have never been able to take estrogen before because it might aggravate such preexisting medical conditions as gallbladder disease, liver disease, a certain kind of hypertension, and clotting problems can safely take it now. That's because a brand-new method of delivering the hormone—the transdermal patch, which is worn like a Band-Aid and delivers estrogen directly through the skin into the bloodstream—bypasses the digestive system and so eliminates any adverse effects on these conditions.

That leaves only a tiny number of women—those with a history of uterine cancer or estrogen-dependent breast cancer—who still can't always take the hormone safely.

STOP WORRYING

The consensus of opinion today among experts, including myself, is that if you need the benefits of estrogen after menopause, you should certainly take it and stop worrying about it. If you have symptoms and bodily changes that prevent you from functioning normally, don't let your fears or your friends talk you out of ERT. If you follow the guidelines detailed here, it won't harm you and it can dramatically improve the quality of your life. It can add years to your life and well-being of your body.

NOT EVERY WOMAN NEEDS IT

The fact that estrogen therapy is safe today doesn't mean that every woman in this world should take it. Many women don't need it. And some won't take it even if they do. Others can manage without it, perhaps helped by one of the alternatives described in this book. Many women require only short-term help from estrogen, just long enough for their bodies to adjust to the changes in hormone levels that occur at menopause. Others may need years, perhaps a lifetime, of hormone replacement therapy if they are going to spend the next third of their lives in good functioning condition.

Mrs. G., whom we talked about before, is a good example of a woman who probably should take long-term estrogen because of the likelihood of developing the most serious consequences of estrogen deficiency. Her slight build, her early menopause, and her family history give her more chance of developing osteoporosis, heart disease, and serious sexual difficulties, all of which can be safely countered by estrogen replacement.

But another of my patients, Mrs. J., needed to take oral estrogen/progesterone for only about three years until her hot flashes and insomnia subsided. After that, she got along very well with the occasional use of vaginal estrogen cream (a form of ERT), which kept her sexually functional.

Ms. F., on the other hand, decided against taking hormones altogether. Her hot flashes and other symptoms were very mild and hardly bothered her. She had menopause at age 59, which meant she wouldn't develop symptomatic osteoporosis or heart disease at an early age, and as a widow with no sexual partner, she isn't concerned about her ability to have intercourse.

WHO NEEDS ERT?

You should consider ERT if you and your doctor have found no other way to cope effectively with the following problems at or after menopause:

Severe symptoms

About 75 percent of women have menopausal symptoms such as hot flashes, sleepless nights, strange skin sensations, mood swings, and palpitations. For some women, these symptoms are insignificant. For others, they are manageable. But many women's lives are made miserable by them.

If you have menopausal manifestations that are severe enough to affect the way you live your life, I suggest you take charge of the situation. It makes no sense to suffer, thinking you have no safe alternative, when help is out there. You are an excellent candidate for ERT and today, unless you have had estrogen-dependent cancer, there's no reason you can't take it. Try the nondrug therapies first, but remember, if they don't do the job, that there is nothing yet discovered that compares with estrogen's effectiveness in relieving these symptoms. See Chapter 5 for more information about how it works.

Osteoporosis

Four out of every 10 women develop symptomatic osteoporosis. If you are in this group, ERT is essential. One of the most serious effects of a diminished estrogen supply is deterioration of bone mass, which can result in bones that fracture easily and is responsible for the plight of all the old (and not-so-old) women you know who are suffering from broken hips, fractured arms, and bent backs.

Until menopause, estrogen helps maintain strong bones. Then, as it diminishes, there is a rapid depletion of bone mass, *no matter how much calcium you consume or how much exercise you get*. If you are a prime candidate for osteoporosis, all the calcium in the world won't prevent fragile bones eventually without the help of estrogen.

Osteoporosis is not entirely reversible. Therefore, if you are susceptible, you must prevent the inevitable excessive bone loss before it begins. Because ERT is the single most effective way to do this—in fact, the *only* way —it's time to forget the old wives' tales and seriously consider it. See Chapter 9 for more facts about your bones and their future. Use the checklist to determine whether you are a likely candidate for brittle bones.

Sexual difficulties

You will almost certainly be forced to give up comfortable sexual intercourse 5, 10, or maybe 15 years after menopause because it will simply become too uncomfortable—or perhaps even impossible—if you don't replace your estrogen. (Yes, vaginal estrogen cream *is* ERT and some of the hormone is absorbed into the general circulation just like any other kind of ERT.)

Painful sex is one of the most common and distressing problems women suffer within a few years of losing their major source of estrogen. It's also the most likely, after hot flashes, to send them to their gynecologists. They are usually astonished, however, to discover that what they thought was their own unique problem is virtually universal.

The vast majority of women find intercourse distinctly uncomfortable within 5 or 10 years after menopause, even if they use lubricants and continue to have regular sexual activity (which does help). Because of the degenerative changes from lack of estrogen, vaginal tissues shrink, becoming dry, irritable, rigid, easily injured, and susceptible to vaginal infections. Lubricants compensate for a while— forever for a few lucky women—but if you're typical you'll need more help than that.

Because estrogen replacement therapy is the only way to rejuvenate these delicate tissues, it warrants consideration even if you decide not to go that route. Chapter 7 will discuss this situation further.

Recurring urinary infections

If you've been finding yourself getting one urinary infection after another, blame this problem, too, on a reduced level of circulating estrogen. Just like the vagina, the tissues lining the urethra gradually shrink and dry, making them susceptible to bacteria and other organisms. Many measures can help to prevent and banish the infections, but only ERT will restore the tissues to a more youthful and infection-resistant state. You can get my advice and the remedies for this typical menopausal problem in Chapter 8.

Early menopause

If you have your menopause—your very last menstrual period—in your 30s or early 40s, you should definitely consider ERT unless there is a very good reason for you not to have it. Because you will be living without estrogen for 10 or 15 years more than the average woman, you'll have an unfortunate head start on the long-term consequences of estrogen deficiency: osteoporosis, sexual and urinary problems, as well as a higher risk of cardiovascular disease.

Instant menopause

If you have instantaneous menopause because your ovaries are damaged or surgically removed before their time, you'll probably have the most severe menopausal symptoms. That's why your doctor will almost invariably prescribe ERT at least for the short term (up to five years or so), unless you have had an estrogen-dependent malignancy.

If you are not taking estrogen and are having hot flashes or other symptoms that make you miserable, be sure your doctor is aware of the new methods of taking ERT that now make it safe even for that small subgroup of women who were formerly denied its benefits because of such ailments as gallbladder or liver disease. You can now take it without the possible side effects (see Chapter 12).

A MAJOR FRINGE BENEFIT: YOUNGER SKIN

There are some significant and occasionally very dramatic fringe benefits of estrogen replacement therapy. For one, women who take ERT definitely tend to look younger than their years. Their skin remains smoother, moister, oilier, and more flexible—in other words, younger. Estrogen won't stop the clock or affect the normal aging of the skin, but it influences the processes affecting the skin that are under this female hormone's specific control (see Chapter 10 for details).

That doesn't mean you should take estrogen for cosmetic purposes alone. It is a drug and should be treated with respect and caution, taken only when needed. But your skin may well be the beneficiary.

THE OTHER FRINGE BENEFITS

There are other side effects of ERT that can be considered benefits. For example, estrogen helps to maintain the firmness and strength of the body's muscle tissue. It keeps your hair stronger and your breasts firmer. There is even some evidence that it helps to alleviate arthritic pain in only a couple of weeks. A brand-new study conducted in The Netherlands even shows that women who take estrogen have a significantly lower incidence of rheumatoid arthritis.

WHAT'S GOING ON?

Menopause used to be a secret, something women didn't care to think about or discuss until they had to. Women knew remarkably little about this natural life event and so they often had no idea whether what was going on was common or uncommon, normal or abnormal.

But today, many women want to know exactly how their bodies function. With the new openness about formerly private areas of life, they are eager to educate themselves, to find out about this normal female biological process with its universals and variables so they can deal with it intelligently. The purpose of this book is give you all of the available facts about what is happening to you now, plus the options for coping with its effects on your body.

GOING FOR IT

Growing numbers of women today are intensely interested in fitness and health and determined to remain active and involved. We are living longer than ever before and there's no reason not to do it in the best possible physical condition. Today a newborn girl can expect to live to 79.5 years, and a woman who has reached 50 in good health may live a lot longer than that. Her life expectancy is about 92. What this means is that most of us at menopause have at least a third of our lives before us.

It is my opinion that it is not fair to require any of us to spend that valuable third of our lives without the benefit of the female hormones our bodies no longer produce—if we need their help.

THE WORLD AROUND US

Society has not been kind to postmenopausal women. It has generally found them ludicrous, archaic, and quite dispensable. Partly that's because menopause is rather new to us. Earlier in history, women rarely lived past menopause and when they did, they turned into old ladies whose purpose was to bake cookies, care for the grandchildren, and mind their own business.

And partly women at this time of their lives have been put down and devalued because the rules and opinions of our society have basically been *man*-made—with female acquiescence. Women have only recently begun to assert themselves, demanding to be treated equally and as people rather than possessions. Men have always made the decisions about the desirability, the attractiveness, the usefulness of women, placing little value on those who no longer had functioning reproductive systems.

As attitudes change, midlife is becoming viewed as a

second life, a chance for reassessment, stretching, growing. Most women today have many interests and don't have time to flutter uselessly around their empty nests when their children leave. They don't fall into disrepair and housedresses, get fat and passive, nor do they lose their femininity and sexuality. As a matter of fact, this is a time for many of us to feel reenergized and renewed by the opportunity to begin a whole new phase of life, often with fewer responsibilities, more time, experience, money, opportunity, and vigor.

That means more of us are greeting midlife, if not with total delight, then with acceptance and serenity, as a time of life when many problems have been resolved, identities have been established, primary responsibilities are fewer, and more pleasures can be savored.

In fact, these are often the best years of our lives.

WHO CARED ABOUT MENOPAUSE?

Amazingly little hard research was ever done on the subject of menopause until only a decade or so ago. This important phase of every woman's life has always been sadly neglected for several reasons. For one thing, it is not a life-threatening disease, or even a disease at all. For another, many of the discomforts a woman may experience when she's going through it do eventually disappear.

But mostly, I think, menopause has been neglected because it is strictly a *woman's* problem. Men don't go through menopause—the idea of a true male menopause is a highly exploited myth. If men did have a menopause and quit producing testosterone, the major hormone responsible for their maleness, is it possible to imagine they would not make every effort to replace it? If it was shown to be safe, are there any intelligent men who savor life who wouldn't take hormone pills?

Besides, virtually all physicians and researchers are men, the very people who need not be concerned with menopause and who may indeed feel threatened by it. Menopause has not been a subject that has warranted concentrated attention from them. Instead, it has often been perceived as a rather amusing and trivial problem, something neurotic women without much else to do made an inordinate fuss about.

But now, with greater numbers of women entering medicine and the demands of women to be treated equally and seriously, plus the more enlightened attitudes of many male physicians, we're already seeing much more attention paid to all of the problems that are exclusively female.

STILL ANOTHER REASON

Another cause for increased interest in the health and happiness of women after midlife is the aging of our population. There are more than 40 million women over the age of 50 in the United States, with 3,500 women joining the group every day. Because most of us will live several more decades, it makes economic, medical, and common sense to take us seriously.

THE SMART WOMAN'S GUIDE TO
MENOPAUSE AND ERT

This book, for intelligent women who have searched
for a thorough and complete guide to menopause and estrogen replacement therapy, is the first to be written by an
expert in the field. We hope you will find the answers to
every question you have ever wanted to ask about this
normal physiological occurrence and its effects on your
body.

Can you prepare for a healthy menopause? To a degree, you can. You can eat properly, exercise enough, quit
smoking, investigate your family's medical history, and
get regular medical checkups, especially if anything seems
at all out of the ordinary.

Most of all, you can learn everything you can about
what's going to happen when your ovaries go out of business. What you learn on these pages will affect the quality
of your life for the rest of your years.

This book is not an argument for taking estrogen, but
for taking action to help yourself if you need it. Suffering
is out of style. Go for it!

2

Is Estrogen Safe?

If estrogen replacement therapy can preserve your bones and your sex life, turn hot flashes and insomnia into memories, and do other wonderful things, why doesn't every woman take it? One obvious answer is that every woman doesn't require it. The other is that there has been serious concern about its safety.

Today we know that estrogen replacement therapy *is* safe *if* it is used correctly. ERT today is very different from the therapy prescribed even a decade ago. Our knowledge has vastly increased since then and techniques have been greatly refined. Today's ERT, according to virtually all of the recent and most respected studies, has been shown not only to be remarkably effective but also remarkably safe.

We're going to give you an overview of ERT's current safety record, starting with the cancer scares of the 1970s, and we hope to answer every one of your most pressing questions. The details will follow later as we discuss each subject. We'll talk about estrogen's effect on uterine and breast cancer, heart disease, clotting problems, gallbladder disease, liver disease, fibroids, hypertension—and every other possible link between ERT and your health.

This is the first guidebook to menopause that discusses all the issues about ERT, pro and con, presenting a balanced view of potential problems and benefits. When you've got all the facts, you can decide from a position of knowledge whether or not you wish to use estrogen.

THE BIG ESTROGEN SCARE

Estrogen was hailed in the 1960s as a miracle medication that could keep you young forever, and many doctors prescribed huge daily doses for any woman who asked for it, often starting long before menopause and recommending continuation for life.

Then in 1975, researchers linked it with uterine cancer, reporting that women who took estrogen were four to eight times more likely to develop this cancer than women who did not.

When the bad news hit the headlines, the use of estrogen immediately and precipitously declined. If women were taking hormones, they quit. If they weren't, they certainly weren't going to start now. In any case, their doctors wouldn't prescribe ERT, even for women in desperate need of it. Estrogen was declared dangerous and that was that, no matter how miserable a woman might be without it. Unfortunately, many women were extremely miserable because there were no satisfactory therapeutic alternatives.

ERT MAKES A COMEBACK

But estrogen has made a comeback and virtually every knowledgeable specialist prescribes it again. That's because new research has found that **ERT is safe when used correctly in the new medically approved way.** You are actually *less* likely to get cancer if you've taken hormones than if you have taken nothing at all. Besides, you are *less* likely to have a heart attack and your life expectancy can be significantly longer.

Using estrogen properly means taking it in low doses (never in the large doses prescribed before) and combined with progesterone for part of every month.

There's always somebody (or her doctor) who still hasn't heard the word and takes estrogen without countering it with progesterone. In fact, a survey made by the pharmaceutical industry reported that, even by mid-1985, progesterone was prescribed with estrogen only 25 percent of the time!

But the rule is: Unless you have had a hysterectomy, you *must* take progesterone when you take estrogen. There is no other safe option.   And even if you have had

a hysterectomy, taking progesterone is still good for your
health.

Using Estrogen Correctly

Using estrogen correctly means it must be:
- Taken in low doses—1.25 mg or less per day of conjugated estrogen (Premarin) or the equivalent amount of other estrogens.
- Combined for part of each month with progesterone—if you have a uterus. Even if you don't, progesterone should still be part of your monthly regime because it will probably protect you against breast cancer.
- Individualized for each woman, because every woman's estrogen sensitivity is different.
- Monitored by regular and thorough gynecological examinations.

Chapter 12 will give you all the details about how to take ERT safely.

Now let's talk about what we know about estrogen and your health.

ESTROGEN AND UTERINE CANCER

There was validity in the early reports of increased incidence of cancer of the uterus among women who took estrogen, even though the studies themselves were flawed. In the 1960s and early 1970s, estrogen was often prescribed in huge doses and "unopposed," which means it was given alone without progesterone, the other major female hormone. This practice did have the potential of causing problems. Here's why.

Estrogen itself does not cause cancer. It is *not* a carcinogen. However, if it is not used correctly, it can cause endometrial hyperplasia, which is an excessive buildup or proliferation of the cells of the uterine lining. This is not cancer. However, among certain women who are predisposed toward cancer of the uterus, hyperplasia can go on to become cancer *if* it is neglected.

That's why it is *essential* to take estrogen in low doses and to use progesterone as well. Low doses and progesterone for a sufficient number of days a month prevent the lining from building up enough to become hyperplastic.

Uterine cancer *always* goes through a hyperplastic stage, though every case of hyperplasia does not turn into cancer even if it isn't treated (just as every rectal polyp doesn't become malignant). Nevertheless, it must not be ignored.

Hyperplasia provides clear warnings: It causes bleeding at unscheduled times and it may produce very heavy menstrual periods before menopause. If you go to a good gynecologist whenever you have irregular or extraheavy bleeding, you will be tested for hyperplasia with a D&C or aspirator. (Do not settle for a Pap test, which may not pick up this condition.)

If tests show you have hyperplasia *(which is a possibility even when you are not taking estrogen therapy),* the best treatment is a few months of progesterone alone to get rid of the excessive buildup of lining. See pages 190 and 193 for more about this.

Incidentally, hyperplasia and nonmalignant fibroid tumors—not cancer—are the most common reasons for hysterectomies. Much of this surgery is totally unnecessary, however, because *early endometrial hyperplasia is almost invariably reversible*. It rarely fails to respond dramatically to treatment with progesterone.

Hyperplasia occurs in about 2 percent of women taking estrogen without progesterone, and occasionally even among those who do take progesterone because they are especially responsive to estrogen and require larger-than-average progesterone doses each month. For this reason, monitoring and individual adjustment of doses are essential elements in keeping ERT absolutely safe.

Valid warnings

Because the huge doses of unopposed estrogen casually given in the 1960s and most of the 1970s sometimes did cause hyperplasia, which was occasionally allowed to go on to become cancer, it was certainly right that women should be warned of the potential danger. At that time, the invaluable role of progesterone was not widely recognized.

Nevertheless, the estrogen scare was a tragedy for women who suffered acutely distressing symptoms and serious disabling disorders that couldn't be helped any other way.

How today's ERT keeps you safe

Estrogen, whether it's manufactured by your own body or taken by way of pill, patch, or vaginal cream, has the job of thickening the endometrium, the lining of the uterus. Progesterone's role, on the other hand, is to precipitate the shedding of that thickened lining. **When suf-ficient progesterone is given each month along with a minimal dose of estrogen, there is no buildup of tissue that could lead to cancer.** Even ERT's most vociferous critics now agree that this is true.

What's more, when you take ERT this way, you are *less* likely to develop cancer of the uterus than women who have never gone anywhere near a hormone pill.

Can hormones stimulate a cancer already there?

Though it won't initiate cancer, estrogen *can* accelerate the growth of a cancer that may already have developed in your uterus. This may not be a disadvantage, however, because it can mean a diagnosis can be made more quickly. Uterine cancer is a rare disease and, unless it is neglected, very few die from it. The reason so few women die of this cancer is that it is so easily detected. It almost invariably reveals itself by bleeding, which means it can be picked up very early in its development. And if it bleeds sooner because of estrogen supplements, it is likely to get earlier attention.

However, estrogen would *never* knowingly be given in a case of endometrial cancer and it is always withheld after the cancer is removed.

How we know it's safe

Many major studies have confirmed the safety of estrogen when it's properly used. Most notable perhaps was a study by Dr. R. Don Gambrell, Jr., of the Medical College of Georgia. Gambrell's study, reported in 1983, was the largest of its kind and covered 8,000 patient years. It clearly demonstrated that the incidence of uterine cancer among women who took estrogen with progesterone was only *half* that of women who took no hormones at all.

My own long-term study, published in *Obstetrics and Gynecology* in 1979, was the first really scientific study of estrogen replacement ever made. It was controlled, prospective, and double-blind. Its purpose was to identify the long-term effects of ERT after 10 years of therapy. We compared women taking estrogen/progesterone with women taking placebos (sugar pills). Over 400 female patients at Goldwater Memorial Hospital in New York City were screened for a final selection of 168. Hospitalized for unrelated chronic diseases, the women were constantly available for careful monitoring in a controlled environment.

Both doctors and patients were unaware of which patients received which medication, and the code would not be broken for 10 years. Before the study began and every six months thereafter, each woman was examined and tested.

After 10 years, the results were identified. They showed a positive and protective effect when estrogens were combined with progesterone. In spite of the facts that higher dosages of hormones were used in the study than are normally taken by menopausal women today and that the therapy continued much longer than most women use it, there were *no* cases of endometrial *or* breast cancer among the women treated with ERT. In the placebo group, however, there was one endometrial cancer and four breast cancers during the 10 years, closely matching the national average for this age group.

Other recent studies show the same results. At King's College School of Medicine in London, Dr. Malcolm I. Whitehead, one of the leading authorities in this sophisticated field, performed endometrial biopsies on thousands of women who were taking estrogen/progesterone therapy. Reported in *Tutorials in Medicine* in 1986, his study found that sufficient progesterone prevents hyperplasia (and therefore cancer) in *all* cases. The vast majority of women will develop no hyperplasia on 5 mg of progesterone for 10 days each month or 10 mg for 7 days, while a few highly susceptible women require a higher dosage. **In other words, hyperplasia and uterine cancer are completely preventable on ERT.**

ESTROGEN AND BREAST CANCER

Because estrogen influences breast tissue, there has always been concern that it could initiate malignancies. It was suspect too because it can speed up the growth of estrogen-dependent cancers that already exist.

However, many scientific studies show no link between ERT and breast cancer, and others present clear evidence that ERT actually helps to prevent it. **Today we know that estrogen does not cause breast cancer and that, when you take low-dose estrogen combined with progesterone, your chances of developing this cancer are significantly less than they would be without the hormones.**

How we know it's safe

The Boston Collaborative Drug Surveillance Study in 1973 followed over 5,000 women on oral contraceptives (which always contain *far* more estrogen than ERT), and found there were fewer cases of breast malignancies among these women than those in a control group.

A second study by the same team, reported in 1974, compared over 5,000 women, ages 45 through 69, who had been admitted into the hospital for breast masses, against over 4,000 comparable women who were admitted for other reasons. Each group contained exactly the *same* percentage of women who had been on ERT, indicating no link between the hormone and cancer.

Our own study at New York's Goldwater Memorial Hospital of 168 women, half on estrogen/progesterone and the other half on placebos, indicated that ERT is *more* than neutral—it is actually protective.

Although the expected rate over a decade in this age group would be four or possibly five cases, there were *no* cases of breast cancer among the estrogen users while there were four cases among the control group who took the placebos.

The most recent and the largest important study of breast cancer and estrogen therapy was done by Dr. R. Don Gambrell, Jr., of the Medical College of Georgia. (This was the same research that investigated the possible link with endometrial cancer.) Gambrell studied 5,563 postmenopausal women for seven years.

His work showed that (1) *women on estrogen alone had a lower incidence of breast cancer than women who took no hormones;* and (2) *women on both estrogen and progesterone had an incidence even lower than that.* This led Gambrell to state that "combined estrogen/progesterone treatment significantly decreases the risk for breast cancer."

The Odds for Breast Cancer

These are the facts about mammary cancer:

- Breast cancer is the most common kind of cancer among women (though lung cancer is now the prime cause of death).

- It is rare before 30 and becomes more prevalent with age.

- One in every 11 women will have it during her lifetime.

- Those women most likely to contract it are those with a strong family history of breast cancer. Women whose mothers had it have a risk five times higher than normal.

- Though women with cystic mastitis or other benign lumps have been thought to be at greater risk, their chances of getting breast cancer seem to be no higher than anyone else's. Because of the multiple cysts, however, new lumps can be missed more easily during the examination.

- The risk of breast cancer rises somewhat if you reached puberty early and/or had menopause late.

- This is also true if you have never had children. Conversely, you have *less* risk if you had your first child at an early age, before 25. And the younger you were at your first pregnancy and the more pregnancies you've had, the better.

- Your risk also decreases if you have breast-fed your children.

Is it or isn't it estrogen-dependent?

It is absolutely essential to know whether an existing breast malignancy is or isn't dependent on estrogen for its growth.

ERT must never be given to anyone with an existing estrogen-dependent cancer because, although it was not responsible for initiating it, it can make this kind of cancer grow more rapidly. In fact, the ovaries and other hormone-producing glands may be removed and estrogen blockers prescribed to reduce estrogen production to as close to zero as possible to starve any undiscovered cancer cells.

For the same reason, it is best to avoid estrogen— except perhaps on a very short-term basis for extremely uncomfortable symptoms—if you have a strong family history of this disease.

On the other hand, breast cancer that is *non*-estrogen-dependent—the kind most common after menopause— will often shrink when the hormone is taken and so women are frequently treated with estrogen after surgery to help prevent a recurrence.

Women who develop breast cancer *before* menopause almost always have the estrogen-dependent type. It is a disease of the reproductive years.

Women who develop it *after* menopause, especially five or more years later, almost always have the non-estrogen-dependent type.

The importance of breast exams

Women over 50 account for about two thirds of the cases of breast cancer, so breast examination becomes more important than ever. It's actually easier to examine your breasts at this age because they become less fibrous and dense after menopause.

Remember to examine yourself at least once a month, just after your periods if you still have them or at the same time every month if you don't. See your doctor every six months for a professional examination. If you are in a high-risk group, it may be wise to see the doctor more often.

Keep in mind you are looking for a lump you haven't felt before. Every breast has lumps and bumps and it's not easy for a nonprofessional to distinguish between them. But usually a bump that is tender, quite movable, and soft is merely a swollen gland. A very hard, small lump, rather like a hard pea, is more likely to be the troublesome variety. But don't make the decision yourself—check out every new lump with your doctor.

Mammography is essential

You should routinely have mammography—breast examination by X ray—once a year if you're over 45, even more often if you are at high risk. Mammography can pick up undiscovered early cancer that cannot be felt and it is absolutely essential over the age of 50. It is especially useful if you have cystic fibrous disease or very large breasts, neither of which is thought to cause a higher incidence of breast cancer but which can make examination for new lumps very difficult.

The new mammography machines emit very low doses of radiation and are no longer to be feared as carcinogenic themselves. Just make sure the machine used for your examination is one of the new ones that require no more than a total of 0.6 roentgens of radiation for the four X ray exposures you'll need.

There are two types of cancer in the breast: One is glandular, the other ductile. The glandular type, which is more likely to be estrogen-dependent, usually produces the tiny pealike lumps, very small, very hard, and felt more easily. The kind that occurs in the ducts can't be felt so early because the ducts give them room to expand surreptitiously. Mammography can pick up these ductile tumors years before they'd ever become evident any other way.

ESTROGEN AND YOUR HEART

Can estrogen keep you alive longer? There is growing evidence that it can by improving the cardiovascular system and protecting you against heart disease. **Women who take estrogen tend to live significantly longer than those who don't.**

At least seven major studies strongly support a beneficial effect of estrogen on the heart. The most widely reported was made by Dr. Trudy L. Bush and colleagues for the National Institutes of Health's National Heart, Lung, and Blood Institute, and published in the *Journal of The American Medical Association* in 1983. This research followed 2,269 women, aged 40 to 69, for an average of 5.6 years to find out whether those women who took estrogen after menopause lived longer than those who didn't.

They did. The death rate for the estrogen users was only a third as high as nonusers.

The most pronounced difference in life span was among women whose ovaries had been surgically removed before menopause. These are women whose risk of heart disease soars because they lose their major supply of estrogen so early. The death rate among the estrogen users in this group was almost *10 times lower* than that of the nonusers.

Dr. Brian E. Henderson, Director of the University of Southern California Comprehensive Cancer Center in Los Angeles, recently reported the results of a longitudinal health study of 435 deaths among 7,610 women in a Southern California retirement community. Women who had used ERT showed a 16 percent reduction in mortality from all causes compared with women who never used it at all.

"About three-quarters of this decline," stated Dr. Henderson, "was due to the reduction in the death rate from acute myocardial infarction among women who had used estrogen . . . even in the presence of other known risk factors."

But the results of two studies that were reported simultaneously in the *New England Journal of Medicine* in 1985 flatly contradict one another concerning the effects of estrogen therapy on heart disease, thoroughly confusing the medical community. One reported that estrogen raises the risk of heart attack, while the other found that it significantly lowers it. The research showing a drop in risk, however, studied 10 times the number of women as the other and did not include oral-contraceptive users among its subjects.

When it comes to hearts, women are the tops

Women have a clear edge over men before age 45 and heart attacks for them are an uncommon occurrence. According to the National Heart Institute, men from the ages of 30 to 39 have 20 times more myocardial infarctions than women in the same age range. From 40 to 49, men outnumber women seven to one. The ratio is five men to one woman from ages 50 to 53. But after 54, women quickly catch up to men and start having just as many heart attacks.

Obviously, young women have protection that men (and older women) don't have. Scientists have long suspected that the reason women live longer than men has something to do with their hormones, especially estrogen.

Why? Nobody knows for sure, but the protection almost certainly comes from estrogen's ability to increase the level of high-density lipoproteins (HDLs), the good lipids, in the blood and with them the protection against cardiovascular disease. It also decreases the low-density lipids (LDLs), the harmful blood fats. The HDLs carry the plaque formed by cholesterol and triglycerides away from artery walls, while the LDLs do the opposite. Dr. Bush's study showed a 10 percent rise in HDLs for women on estrogen and an 11 percent reduction in LDLs, a wonderful combination.

Estrogen is also thought to help maintain the elasticity and general health of the arteries, making them more efficient in their job of pumping blood to and from the heart.

Losing your edge with early menopause

Unfortunately, early menopause changes your odds. If you have menopause before 40 or have your ovaries removed before your supply of estrogen peters out on its own, your chances of heart disease are greatly increased.

Within only five years (if you don't take estrogen), you have the very same risk of heart disease and heart attacks as men. (Obviously, this doesn't apply when only one ovary has been removed, leaving the other to continue making hormones.)

Does estrogen encourage clots?

It is true, as charged, that among women who take oral contraceptives, estrogen does encourage blood clots and therefore heart attacks and strokes. However, it is *not* true among women on postmenopausal low-dose ERT.

What's the difference? All oral contraceptives, even today's low-dose birth-control pills, contain far higher amounts of estrogen than ERT.

High-dose estrogen (2.5 mg or more of conjugated estrogen per day or the equivalent amount of other estrogens) decreases the anticlotting factors of the blood, which means clots will form more readily. For this reason, women should go off The Pill by 35 when this may start to become a problem. It's the same reason they shouldn't take The Pill if they smoke. Smoking also reduces the anticlotting factors, besides compromising the vascular bed and constricting circulation.

However, low-dose estrogen—0.625 mg or less of conjugated estrogen a day or the equivalent amount of other estrogens—has *no* effect on the anticlotting factors for virtually all women. That means it is quite safe to take even if you have varicose veins.

If you have a history of thrombophlebitis or thromboemboli, however, especially if you are very heavy, ERT may not be advisable for you because you are especially susceptible to clotting and you shouldn't risk even the most minute effect. If you need estrogen badly, your doctor may prescribe a low dose, then test your blood to see if the anticlotting factors have remained normal.

In any case, vaginal estrogen cream and the new transdermal patch method of ERT seem to eliminate the possibility of clotting problems, whether you are at high risk or not. So, if there is any question of complications with oral estrogen, the cream or the patch is the route to take.

Does progesterone neutralize the benefits?

Adding progesterone to ERT has many terrific advantages, such as preventing cancer, but it can also discourage HDLs, the benevolent blood lipids that protect your arteries. So medical researchers worry whether it will neutralize the good effects of estrogen on lipoproteins and therefore on heart disease.

The progesterone in oral contraceptives does affect the lipoproteins adversely, radically lowering the levels of the beneficial HDLs.

But the form of progesterone used for ERT, medroxyprogesterone acetate, is different. It affects blood lipids only minimally. An added attraction is that this progesterone's effects on blood fats are dose-related. The newest research indicates that ERT's tiny amounts rarely affect blood fats adversely and so won't neutralize the beneficial effects of estrogen.

ESTROGEN AND HYPERTENSION

In about 1 out of every 20 women, oral estrogen causes a release of two enzymes, renin and angiotensin, from the kidneys, sometimes precipitating a rise in blood pressure. However, there's no need to go back to hot flashes, insomnia, or painful sex. Take your estrogen by vaginal cream or use the new transdermal skin patch, which doesn't have the same effect on the kidneys.

ESTROGEN AND GALLSTONES

ERT taken by mouth can raise your risk of symptomatic gallstones, probably because it tends to thicken and concentrate the bile produced by the liver. That's why many women with gallbladder disease had to suffer postmenopausal problems without help from hormones. Here, too, if you take your estrogen via vaginal cream or the transdermal patch, you will rule out this problem. By avoiding the "hepatic first-pass effect" because it is not ingested, it does not affect the bile and therefore does not promote the formation of gallstones.

ESTROGEN AND LIVER IMPAIRMENT

The liver is responsible for metabolizing the estrogen that passes through it. When it is damaged, it may not do this job properly and so the hormone may actually become toxic. Oral estrogen should never be taken if your liver function is impaired. However, vaginal estrogen cream and transdermal estrogen do not send the hormone through the liver and once again solve a major problem.

ESTROGEN AND DIABETES

Low-dose estrogen seldom affects sugar metabolism, even though the high doses in birth-control pills can definitely throw it off. So ERT is almost always safe for diabetics. Nevertheless, your physician should keep an eye on your blood-sugar tests.

ESTROGEN AND FIBROIDS

Fibroid tumors are probably the most common reason why doctors have warned women against taking estrogen. But times have changed. Today, estrogen doses are so small that they rarely affect these benign muscle tumors that are almost invariably found in the uterine walls of women over 40.

If fibroids become very large, they may bleed profusely or impinge on the territory of nearby organs such as the bladder. Because they are under estrogen control, they grow under the influence of the hormone and usually shrink as this hormone gradually peters out with menopause.

So, is it safe or wise to take estrogen after menopause if you have fibroids? In most cases, yes. The amount of estrogen in low-dose ERT today is much less than you used to make in your own ovaries, and it is rarely enough to make fibroids grow. Occasionally, though, it does. If that's the case for you and your fibroids are already large, then you'd be best advised to discontinue the estrogen.

As you can see, estrogen replacement therapy is now considered safe when it's used correctly. So our advice is: If you need estrogen's help, don't be afraid of it. Do it right and it's not going to hurt you.

ON TO YOUR PHYSIOLOGY

Now let's talk about the changes in your body at the time of menopause so you can decide intelligently what you're going to do about them.

3

How Your Body Prepares for Menopause

MENOPAUSE IS A MYSTERY to an astonishing number of women who haven't thought much about it before, but it is a natural and normal life event that happens to every woman on earth who lives long enough to experience it.

To understand menopause, you have to recognize the important role estrogen has played throughout your reproductive life, starting with puberty.

When your reproductive years are finished and your body starts getting ready for menopause, it goes through a changeover. You gradually stop ovulating and your ovaries slow down their production of progesterone and estrogen, the two major female hormones. This time of your life is called *perimenopause*, a trying time for many women because what happens now is often unpredictable, and if you're like most of my patients, you're never sure what's normal and what isn't.

Here's a short explanation of what goes on in your body from puberty to menopause. In the next chapter, we'll talk about menopause itself—the time of your life *after* your very last menstrual period.

YOUR REPRODUCTIVE YEARS

Estrogen is the substance that is responsible for turning a little girl's body into a woman's, making conception and pregnancy possible. A few years before menarche (the first menstrual period), a girl's ovaries begin to secrete this important hormone in response to stimulation from the follicle-stimulating hormone (FSH) produced by the pituitary, the master gland. In turn, the FSH release has been turned on by a part of the brain called the hypothalamus which puts out gonadotropin-releasing hormone (GNRH).

A couple of years after starting to produce estrogen, a young girl begins ovulating and becomes fertile. Ovulation then stimulates the production of progesterone, the other major female hormone that together with estrogen is responsible for menstruation.

Every month or so until she reaches menopause—perhaps interrupted by pregnancies—the normal woman goes through a typical menstrual cycle. The hypothalamus begins the cycle by producing gonadotropin-releasing hormone. Stimulated by this hormone, the pituitary gland secretes FSH, which then causes the release of estrogen from the ovaries.

Now the egg follicles start to develop. One of them reaches maturity in about two weeks and the others stop growing. The follicle is ready to ovulate or to release the egg. The pituitary releases a second hormone called luteinizing hormone (LH) in response to the ovaries' peak production of estrogen. The LH causes the egg to be released.

Once ovulation has occurred, the egg drops into the fallopian tube and sets off on its way to the uterus.

Meanwhile, the corpus luteum, the piece of the follicle left behind after the egg is released, takes over an important endocrine function. Within a few days, it produces progesterone, which peaks in several days. This means that in the first part of the cycle, there is a steadily increasing secretion of estrogen from the ovary, and in the second part of the cycle, there is a secretion of *both* estrogen and progesterone from the scar left over from ovulation.

Meanwhile, what is happening back at the lining of the uterus, the endometrium?

The estrogen builds up the endometrium by proliferating the cells into a thickened tissue ready to support a fertilized egg and a developing fetus. When the egg is not fertilized, however, the progesterone breaks this thick lining down into three layers, ready to be shed.

Now menstruation begins—the lining is cleanly and completely sloughed off as a result of progesterone's action and flows out through the opening of the uterus into the vagina, leaving behind a healthy membrane. And the cycle begins again.

This whole cyclical process starts to change as your body approaches menopause.

PERIMENOPAUSE: YOUR BODY GETS READY FOR MENOPAUSE

Perimenopause, the time when your body is preparing for menopause, can be a particularly difficult time for many women, though it rarely lasts longer than a year. You may have competely erratic periods and perhaps some very stressful symptoms, even though for most women the symptoms don't make an appearance until menopause actually happens.

It's important to know that *this is no time to start estrogen replacement therapy* even though you may desperately want it. You're still making estrogen, sometimes just a little, but sometimes an extraordinary amount, as we will explain shortly.

THE PHYSIOLOGICAL CHANGES

About two to four years before you have your very last menstrual period, your menopause, you stop ovulating. Or you produce eggs irregularly or only occasionally. You have depleted all or almost all of your allotted follicles, though your ovaries are continuing to produce estrogen.

On the other hand, because progesterone production is totally dependent on ovulation, that important hormone quits. That's why your periods now may be so erratic. The estrogen continues to build up the endometrium—the uterine lining—but there's no (or only occasional) proges-terone to make it shed on its former monthly schedule.

Now, instead of regular periods, you bleed at unex-pected times as the endometrium comes off whenever it's ready, rarely cleanly and completely.

SIGNS OF PERIMENOPAUSE

When you are in perimenopause, you'll probably skip some periods. Your periods may be days late—or a week early. They may be short or long, scant or heavy, perhaps with clumps of endometrial tissue. Maybe they will start and stop and then start again. They may vanish for several months and then return for several more. Often there's no discernible pattern at all to your menstrual cycle and it varies in almost every possible way. This erratic nonpat-tern, almost a mirror image of what happened in puberty, can be very unsettling.

Perimenopause is brief if you are fortunate, lasting only a few months. The average duration, however, is about a year and it can go on for as long as five or six years.

Some women, the lucky ones, go through no erratic periods at all, but simply stop menstruating one day and that is that.

COULD YOU BE PREGNANT?

It's perfectly normal to skip a period or two or maybe more because your ovaries are winding down and you're not making much progesterone. But there is a remote chance that the skipped periods mean you're pregnant! If there is any possibility that this could be true, check it out with your gynecologist. Ovulation is erratic during perimenopause, and once in a while you may produce a viable egg which may become fertilized. That is why contraception is always advised for at least a year after your last period.

Once your FSH level is above 40 MIU/mL, it would be almost impossible for you to get pregnant. But *almost* is an important word, because there is a chance that even though you haven't been ovulating for months, the high FSH may stimulate the ovaries to send out just one more egg. And that egg may turn into a change-of-life baby!

Whether or not you want to have a baby is a big decision and whatever you conclude requires action now. Go to your doctor and check out your status even if you feel positive you've had menopause.

WHEN DO MENOPAUSAL SYMPTOMS START?

You probably won't have any menopausal symptoms during this preliminary period, the perimenopause. Usually, these begin only after you've stopped menstruating altogether. But in 15 to 20 percent of women the typical menopausal symptoms (see the next chapter), perhaps accompanied by noticeable mood swings similar to premenstrual tension, begin during this time of irregular periods. Though vaginal dryness becomes especially apparent after menopause, it too may start to develop now.

NO ESTROGEN REPLACEMENT NOW!

It is *dangerous* to start estrogen replacement therapy in perimenopause. That's because you may be producing tremendous amounts of estrogen, and by taking even more you may elevate the hormone level to a perilously high level. The huge amounts of estrogen make the uterine lining proliferate quickly. At the same time, you are not ovulating and therefore not producing progesterone, the hormone responsible for getting rid of that built-up lining.

This may sound contradictory until you understand what is happening. As the years go by and you run out of eggs, your ovaries slow down, making less and less estrogen. But the pituitary has no way of knowing that. So when the estrogen reaches a certain level, the pituitary begins to work overtime in a desperate attempt to stimulate the ovaries to get back in business again. It produces huge amounts of FSH and, at the same time, it releases large quantities of luteinizing hormone (LH) to encourage ovulation. The alarm is passed along to the hypothalamus in the brain and it too gets busy, putting out more gonadotropin-releasing hormone.

The normal amount of circulating FSH during the reproductive years is below 40 MIU/mL. Now your FSH could rise to well over 40, sometimes as high as 1,000. Once the FSH level goes up, it usually stays up, perhaps for the rest of your life, though eventually your body adjusts to its presence.

In perimenopause, whatever remaining estrogen-producing cells you still have will respond to the FSH and work at top speed to make more hormone. Besides, a small amount of additional estrogen may be converted by the fat cells from the androgens, the malelike hormones produced by every woman's adrenals.

That's why, paradoxically, your estrogen level may become astronomical at a time when your ovaries are shutting down. Without the progesterone to clean out the built-up lining, you may then go on to develop hyperplasia, an overproliferated endometrium, which could possibly set the stage for cancer if it's allowed to continue to build.

This is why it is crucial that you do not start taking estrogen replacement therapy now.

SHAPING UP YOUR PERIODS WITH PROGESTERONE

If your irregular and erratic periods unnerve you, there is something to be done to get them back on a nice predictable schedule until they decide to desert you forever.

If you take progesterone (alone, never with estrogen) for one week a month, you will have regular periods until you run out of estrogen. Your doctor will have to prescribe it for you, usually in doses of 10 mg per day for seven days.

The progesterone will also make sure your endometrium is cleanly shed each month. It is often prescribed for just that reason. Many women build up so much endometrial tissue at this time that they require the progesterone to prevent or alleviate an abnormally heavy accumulation of lining tissue.

When progesterone is given alone at this time, it can be used, too, as a way to avoid endometrial biopsies. Biopsies every six months or so are the usual way to check out irregular bleeding to be sure it is due to perimenopause and not an abnormal condition. If the monthly progesterone treatment produces regular periods—with no bleeding at other times—your doctor will know all is well. And you won't require another biopsy so soon.

Some women at this stage of reproductive life constantly worry about pregnancy. The monthly progesterone, with its reassuring monthly periods, also eliminates that concern.

Eventually, when you run out of sufficient estrogen to cause the lining to build up every month, your periods will stop even if you continue to take the progesterone.

IT'S TIME TO GO TO THE DOCTOR!

When you start having irregular periods, you *must* see your gynecologist. Do not assume you are about to have menopause, especially if you are below the usual age for it.

The bleeding could be the result of a more serious situation and it requires investigation. Most doctors take a sample of the endometrial lining—an endometrial biopsy —at this time to be sure it is normal. Then if you continue to bleed irregularly, they will test it every six months because there is always a small chance that the bleeding is not caused by perimenopause but by hyperplasia, a polyp, large fibroids, or perhaps another hormonal problem such as hypothyroidism. Cancer, too, is a remote possibility. So don't take chances. Go to the doctor. In most cases, a gynecologist is the best choice.

SYMPTOMS DURING PERIMENOPAUSE

You already know that perimenopause, the time before you have your very last period, is not the time to take estrogen. But what can you do if you're among the 15 or 20 women out of 100 who get hot flashes (heat waves) or other vasomotor menopausal symptoms at this early stage?

If you're lucky, low-dose progesterone (2.5 mg a day) will alleviate them, though it doesn't always help. A long-acting progesterone called Depo-Provera works exceptionally well, eliminating flashes miraculously. But it must be taken by injection (150 mg in water, injected intramuscularly every three months) and, unfortunately, though it may be prescribed for other purposes, it has not yet been approved for this use by the FDA.

TRY VITAMIN E

Happily, daily doses of vitamin E can often do an adequate job of keeping perimenopausal hot flashes under control. Though no one knows exactly how it works—especially since vitamin E is a coenzyme that is not normally manufactured in the human body—it seems to help maintain the estrogen level on a more even keel. Try taking 400 units twice a day and, if necessary, double the dose for a daily total of 1600 units.

For constant and disconcerting PMS-like mood swings, discuss with your doctor whether tranquilizers or mood elevators can be used until the tremendous peaks and valleys of estrogen production have leveled off.

Most important, remember that perimenopause is a transient phase that rarely lasts longer than a year.

MENOPAUSE AT LAST!

Eventually you will have no menstrual periods, erratic or otherwise. When you've had none for 12 consecutive months, you can safely conclude you've reached menopause.

To make sure this is truly the case, especially before prescribing estrogen replacement therapy, your doctor will confirm your status by sending a blood sample out to be analyzed for circulating FSH. A serum FSH level of 40 MIU/ml (2000 picograms) or higher is proof that you've really had menopause.

Why doesn't your physician simply measure your estrogen level? Because the tests for estrogen are extremely inaccurate. They are unnecessary anyway if the FSH test is done. See Chapter 12 for the other essential procedures before starting ERT.

Now, on to menopause.

4

MENOPAUSE: WHAT'S GOING ON?

MENOPAUSE IS your very last menstrual period. It's just one moment in time, a single event in a long physiological process called the climacteric syndrome. This syndrome is a sequence of happenings that may go on for more than 35 years, starting in your late 20s or early 30s when your estrogen production begins to taper off, and ending long after menopause.

The climacteric includes all those years of diminishing estrogen production, both before and after your last period. At one point in the climacteric, when the hormone produced by the ovaries is no longer sufficient to stimulate ovulation and menstrual periods, you have menopause. Meanwhile, the climacteric continues, with the hormone level inexorably diminishing and more changes happening in your body because of it.

The whole process is like puberty in reverse. All the parts and reproductive abilities of your body that once developed in puberty and then were maintained by estrogen now begin to change again as the ovaries gradually give up their dominant role.

WHEN WILL IT HAPPEN?

The average age for menopause, your very last period, is 52, with a normal range of 45 to 55. Some women, of course, have theirs much earlier—or much later. About five out of every hundred women continue to menstruate after 53, some even as late as 60 or more. Approximately eight out of a hundred have menopause before the age of 40.

Your age at menopause is mainly determined by your genes. So, with no outside interference, you will have your last period about the same age as your mother, grandmothers, aunts, and sisters had theirs.

Nobody knows why the ovaries stop producing estrogen at a certain time, but it probably happens when your ovarian follicles are finally depleted. At birth, a female child possesses approximately 400,000 follicles. By the age of 40, the average woman only has 5,000 to 10,000 left and the numbers decline unrelentingly thereafter.

Contrary to what most people think, the age you were

when you had your first period has *no* relationship to the age you'll be at menopause. In fact, there is no correlation at all between these two most important events in your biological history. So whether you begin having periods at 12 or 17 has no bearing on what's going to be.

Of course, you will have menopause *instantly*, from one day to the next, at whatever age you are, if your ovaries are severely damaged or surgically removed before they have stopped making hormones on their own.

THE REASONS FOR EARLY MENOPAUSE

If you are among the 8 percent of women who have spontaneous (that is, nonsurgical) menopause before the age of 40, it's probably because you come from a family that tends to run out of eggs very early. But there are a few other possible, though rare, reasons. Some women inherit an abnormal number of chromosomes and quit making estrogen at a very early age, perhaps even in their 20s. And occasionally a woman suffers from an autoimmune disease, causing her to produce antibodies to her own ovarian tissue.

Women who have had hysterectomies many years before their menopause (but who still have their ovaries) tend to have it earlier than their genes would have dictated. So do women who have had tubal ligations. That's because some blood circulation may have been compromised in the pelvic area as a result of the surgery.

Increasingly common reasons for premature menopause today are chemotherapy and radiation because more and more women now survive cancer. Both treatments can destroy ovarian function and precipitate menopause.

SMOKING: A MAJOR CULPRIT

Heavy smoking can cause you to have menopause before your time! Women who smoke tend to have menopause 5 to 10 years earlier than their nonsmoking relatives. If you are a devotee of cigarettes, the fact that smoking can so seriously affect a normal bodily process should give you yet another reason to reconsider the habit.

THE PROS AND CONS OF EARLY MENOPAUSE

Lots of women are delighted to have an early menopause because it means no more menstrual periods and no more pregnancies. But premature menopause or menopause at the early end of the normal spectrum does have its drawbacks.

The major risk is that you will develop the consequences of estrogen deficiency much sooner than you would have if it had happened later. Your extra years without estrogen give you that much more time to develop some major health problems associated with estrogen deficiency: osetoporosis, vaginal-urinary changes, and cardiovascular disease.

On the other hand, you have less chance of getting ovarian cancer because you have spent fewer years of your life ovulating. (This is the same reason why women who have taken oral contraceptives for any length of time also have a lower incidence of ovarian cancer.)

LATE MENOPAUSE: WHAT'S GOOD ABOUT IT?

If you're among the 5 percent of women who continue to produce enough estrogen for ovulation and menstruation after the age of 53, you have several advantages over those who stop much earlier. That's because the longer you have estrogen circulating throughout the tissues of the body, the longer you are protected against some of the changes that happen when you lose it.

Your estrogen, for example, protects you against cardiovascular disease. It prevents you from developing osteoporosis, giving you stronger bones as "money in the bank" for the future when they won't retain as much calcium as they do now. It helps maintain your youthful appearance. It keeps your vaginal and urinary tissues in good operating condition. Since it takes about 10 years from the time you lose your major source of estrogen until these tissues are seriously affected, you are way ahead if you have a late menopause.

The only real disadvantage of a late menopause is that it puts you at a slightly higher risk for ovarian cancer. That's because the more ovulations you have throughout your lifetime, the more likely you are to develop this kind of cancer. If you are in your 50s and not yet menopausal, most doctors would recommend a thorough physical examination of your ovaries at least once a year, perhaps supplemented by an ultrasound picture, to make certain that all is well. Ovarian cancer produces no symptoms in its early stages.

HOW YOUR BODY CHANGES

Many of the typical changes that start taking place in your body happen to *every* woman at menopause. Every woman stops menstruating and becomes infertile. Every woman's reproductive organs, no longer needed for conception and pregnancy, shrink and change. Every woman's skin, muscles, and bones show the effects of the depletion of the major female hormones she's been producing since puberty.

The ovaries, once the size of a walnut, shrink to about a third of their former size. The flow of mucus from the cervix and vagina gradually wanes. The endometrium thins and shrinks until it finally becomes nonfunctioning. The uterus slowly diminishes from its original size (about as big as your fist and approximately two inches thick) to about a third of its former dimensions.

The walls of the vagina thin out and lose much of their resilience and elasticity. The membrane that lines it becomes thinner because a certain kind of cells, which formed a tough protective layer when estrogen was plentiful, disappear. The distance between the vagina and the urethra becomes shorter, and the urethra's tissues become thinner and more fragile.

The breasts shed their former thick layer of subcutaneous fat and their glandular tissue shrinks because it no longer must be ready to nourish a baby.

Every woman loses much of the fat layer just under the

skin and notices a distinct loss of skin oil and moisture. Muscles tend to lose tone and bone mass diminishes.

The changes that happen to every woman, all of them atrophic in nature, usually start to become evident within about three years after menopause, though sometimes you will notice signs of them even before that.

THE TIMING DIFFERS

Every woman's timetable is different. If your ovaries, along with your adrenal glands and fat tissue, continue to produce some estrogen after menopause—though not enough to sustain ovulation and menstrual periods, of course—these universal changes will occur at a more leisurely pace. At the other extreme, if your ovaries are removed, abruptly and almost completely cutting off your estrogen supply, the changes will occur much more quickly.

THE END OF YOUR REPRODUCTIVE YEARS

When you consider that most of the parts of the female body that alter after menopause are those associated with reproduction, you can understand what is going on. Because your body no longer has to be prepared to respond instantly to the growth and nourishment of a fetus, it returns to a reproductively quiescent state. That's a great relief for many of us and most women today greet the absence of menstrual periods and fertility with equanimity if not joy.

THE VARIABLE CHANGES: WHO GETS WHAT?

There are other common occurrences in a woman's body at menopause, though not everyone experiences them in the same way. These are the responses to the new low levels of female hormones, the "symptoms" of the sharp shift that's taking place rather than changes in body tissues. When the hormonal upheaval stabilizes and the body adjusts, they disappear.

The most common symptom is, of course, the notorious hot flash, the sudden envelopment of the upper body with a wave of heat and perspiration and the subject of many not-very-funny jokes. But there are many other common symptoms: palpitations, insomnia, numbness, pins and needles, crawly skin sensations, strange pains, shortness of breath, dizziness, fatigue, headaches, irritability, and/or depression.

That's quite a long list, but nobody ever has all of them and probably nobody ever has most of them either. Some women never have any. But when you have them, they are not figments of your imagination but real physiological phenomena. They're not harmful, but they can make you pretty uncomfortable and, in some cases, absolutely miserable. Eventually, however, they will pass.

About 1 in every 10 women has no really noticeable outward signs of menopause and wouldn't know anything was happening if she didn't stop having menstrual periods. This is because her production of female hormones diminishes so gradually and gently that her body has time to adjust without stress.

The rest of us, the great majority, will have some of the

symptoms. Most women experience, at the very least, some hot flashes and excessive perspiration, which may not bother them in the slightest but may simply be interesting to observe. But for other women, the flashes, the sweats, and some of the other symptoms may be frequent or severe enough to affect the quality of their lives.

What are you going to do about them? Can you live with them or do you need help? You'll find your alternatives in Chapter 6.

5

Hot Flashes and Other Strange Symptoms

NOBODY CAN PREDICT how you're going to weather menopause because everybody's different. Some women hardly notice the entire phenomenon. They simply stop having menstrual periods and that's that. Others find this is one of the most trying times of their lives, with symptoms that make it impossible for them to function normally. Between the two extremes are the majority of us who have symptoms ranging from insignificant to miserable.

Whatever goes on with you, remember that you are *normal* and that these physiological events are not imaginary. This is a measurable physical happening, the time when your body gradually loses its ability to produce eggs, estrogen, and babies.

WHY THE DIFFERENCES?

Whether or not you develop symptoms at menopause is not under your control, but simply a matter of the inherited rate at which you stop producing estrogen. If you lose estrogen very rapidly, you will probably be seriously affected by your changing hormonal levels. That's why women who lose theirs abruptly because of surgery usually have the worst problems. But if you have lucky genes and lose your ability to make copious estrogen very slowly—and especially if you continue, as many women do, to produce significant estrogen in your adrenals, fat tissue, and even your ovaries—your symptoms will be negligible.

There's nothing superior or inferior about either response. The typical menopausal symptoms such as hot flashes, palpitations, tingling skin, and insomnia don't happen only to unfulfilled discontents, hypochondriacs, or women who have failed to lead healthy, sane, active lives.

As a colleague puts it, "Women who complain about hot flashes are not women who are neurotic—they are women having bad hot flashes. And women who do not complain of hot flashes are not wonderful stoic women of good pioneer stock—they are women who are *not* having bad hot flashes!"

So stop blaming yourself, as so many women do, if

you are overwhelmed by symptoms, and spend your energy instead on helping yourself cope with them.

DON'T PUT UP WITH MISERY

The variable and transient menopausal symptoms such as hot flashes are not dangerous or harmful, no matter how bad they feel. And, except in rare cases, they disappear after a while even if you don't do anything about them.

When they make your life miserable, however, you needn't simply endure them, though an amazing number of women put up with them for months or even years before looking for help. All of the symptoms can be eliminated in very short order by estrogen replacement therapy (ERT), safe for virtually every woman today. If you can't take estrogen or don't want to, there are alternative remedies described in the next chapter that may help. However you decide to do it, fight back!

THE NOTORIOUS HOT FLASH

Of all the variable transient symptoms, the most common is the hot flash (or, if you are British, the hot flush). Flashes can be mild or severe, slightly discomforting or definitely distressing. Sometimes they are even frightening, but they are quite harmless.

Nine out of every ten women have hot flashes or some other vasomotor disturbance. For half of these women, the symptoms are all over within a year. For 30 percent of them, they last up to two and a half years. For the remaining 20 percent, the flashes and/or other vasomotor symptoms hang in for longer than that, maybe 5 or 10 years, sometimes even 20 years. Some unfortunate women—an estimated 2 to 3 percent—have them till the day they die. Because the 1970s were a time when many women gave up estrogen replacement and were afraid to start it because of the reports of a link with cancer, doctors today see an astonishing number of women who had menopause years and years ago, never took estrogen, and are still suffering with heavy flashes.

Many women have only three or four episodes a day and hardly notice them, while others have 30, 40, or even 50 severe hot flashes a day, one right after the other. The flashes are usually at their worst at night.

Hot Flash Facts

• A hot flash is a feeling of intense heat that envelops the body, usually only from the waist up and especially the face and neck. The blood vessels on the skin's surface dilate, causing a rosy flush. In most cases, the flash is accompanied by profuse perspiration. Many women find their bodies and heads become so wet that they have to change all their clothes or even the sheets on the bed, while others merely have to wipe their brows.

Very overweight women tend to have particularly bad flashes, probably because of their greater skin surface and already-stressed circulation.

• A hot flash is often sensed a few seconds before it occurs. You may have "an aura," or an uneasy feeling that tips you off to the impending heat wave.

• The flash is often followed by chills and sometimes intense shivering, along with a feeling of constriction of the skin that may last for a few hours.

• Several studies have shown that skin temperature is measurably elevated during a flash and that there is a 10 to 15 percent increase in pulse rate. These effects start just before the flash occurs.

• Flashes usually last for three to six minutes, though they may last up to an hour.

• Hot sweats, as flashes are called in the vernacular, probably represent the triggering of normal thermal mechanisms at inappropriate times. Your temperature-control mechanism has temporarily gone haywire, making your capillaries dilate and your skin perspire even without a rise in internal or external temperature.

• Some women suffer a variation of hot flashes—they have "cold sweats" which is just what they sound like: chills with profuse perspiration and uncontrollable shivering.

What causes them?

As the years go by and you run out of eggs and estrogen, the pituitary gland starts working desperately to make the ovaries get going again, producing vast amounts of follicle-stimulating hormone (FSH) and luteinizing hormone (LH). It is the heightened level of these pituitary hormones, or perhaps their pulselike bursts, along with the increased activity of a neurotransmitter called norepinephrine in the brain's hypothalamus, that throw the heat-regulating systems off their normal track.

The level of estrogen deficiency at which you're likely to have flashes can differ widely. Some women have no flashes until their estrogen level is very low and their FSH level is extremely high, while others have them at any time during the changing biological procedure.

What triggers flashes?

If you are very susceptible, almost anything can trigger them, especially if they normally raise body temperature and/or dilate the skin's capillaries. For example, a flash may be set off by exercise, external temperature, overwork, excessive clothing, fear, joy, excitement, anxiety. Alcohol and caffeine, both of which cause the capillaries to dilate, will do it too. So will hot drinks and spicy foods.

Although flashes tend to occur less frequently when you are relaxed and rested, they are at their worst at night. We don't know why but it's probably because the hypothalamus responds most vigorously to the super supply of the stimulating hormones when it's in a resting state.

Cooling off flashes

If you're going to get flashes, you'll get them no matter what if you don't take estrogen. But if you take some practical measures, you may ward off a few now and then. For example, because fatigue makes you more susceptible, try to get sufficient rest. Dress in layers so you can remove some clothing when you begin to feel warm. As far as possible, stay clear of emotional upheaval and try to keep

your cool. Give up the drinks and the foods that trigger
the heat. Be sure to eat balanced meals and get adequate
exercise.

OTHER TYPICAL VASOMOTOR SYMPTOMS

This is a time when you may have some other strange
sensations that you may not have associated with menopause. All of them, like flashes, result from vasomotor
instability and are considered hot-flash equivalents.

One of them is palpitations, which are distinct and
rapid heartbeats. They are vasomotor phenomena that are
very common at menopause and do not mean you are
suffering from heart trouble.

You may feel dizzy occasionally. Or you may feel faint
now and then, or get a sensation similar to seasickness.

You may notice peculiar sensations in your arms and
hands, especially your fingers, and these too are vasomotor events. Some women describe them as tingling or pins
and needles, while others get a feeling of numbness that
comes and goes.

Undoubtedly the strangest, and often the most
frightening, menopausal symptom of all is formication, a
crawling feeling over the skin. Luckily this is fairly rare.
One patient recently thought she was having an emotional
breakdown because of these odd sensations and, like
everyone else who gets this one, was enormously relieved
to find out it is a typical, though infrequent, menopausal
occurrence. She was even more relieved when she found
out she could get rid of the crawly feelings with estrogen
replacement.

"DOCTOR, I CAN'T SLEEP!"

Almost every woman suffers from insomnia, minor or major, at this time of hormonal upheaval. And anyone who consistently gets too little sleep feels awful. Sometimes the problem lasts for years.

Some physicians think that sleeping problems are merely a result of hot flashes, that the heat and sweating are responsible for waking you up. It certainly is true that nobody can sleep through a severe hot flash that causes intense heat and so much perspiration that nightclothes and perhaps the sheets and the mattress are soaked. Almost all hot flashes are associated with waking episodes.

But menopausal insomnia is more than that. The hypothalamus controls sleep as well as temperature and hormone production. The insomnia is also caused by changes in sleep patterns and brain waves from the same hypothalamic disturbances that result in the hot flashes and an overstimulated central nervous system. So, between hot flashes and these disturbances, getting enough sleep can become a big problem.

Many women find it hard to fall asleep at night. Others wake up in the middle of the night and toss around for an hour or two. Probably the most common pattern is to wake up very early in the morning, long before you care to, and find it impossible to drop off again. Meanwhile, you worry about how you'll feel all day.

Insomnia is second only to hot flashes as the symptom that propels women to their doctors' offices for help during this period of physiological changeover.

ALL IN YOUR HEAD?

If your emotions seem out of whack around the time of menopause, consider yourself a member of the club. Among the symptoms commonly attributed to this absolutely normal phase of life are depression, irritability, fatigue, tension, instability, and anxiety. Menopause definitely has an emotional component and it is not all in your head. There is a real and measurable physiological aspect to it.

Women have described their feelings as very similar to premenstrual tension. Though it has become unfashionable to blame any mood swings on "the change," it is true that a drop in circulating estrogen *can* affect your emotions. So if you are feeling emotionally fragile, it may make you feel better to know it's not your imagination.

A shift in almost any hormone of any variety, sex-related or not, can affect mood and, in fact, psychological symptoms are often used in diagnosing hormonal imbalances. Estrogen is no exception. Just like the other variable symptoms, the periods of emotional stress occur most often and most noticeably in women whose hormone supply is abruptly or rapidly ended. They also correlate very closely with the fluctuations of hormone levels that occur over and over again during the climacteric.

The emotions are affected by the hypothalamus, the same part of the brain that becomes overactivated and causes flashes. The hypothalamus controls the central nervous system and the activities of many glands that secrete hormones. In addition, the level of circulating estrogen itself affects the way you feel.

IT'S LIKE PREMENSTRUAL TENSION

Premenstrual tension has been shown to correlate with low levels of estrogen and high levels of progesterone just before the menstrual period. It's a time when many women feel irritable, tense, anxious, depressed, and edgy. Then, when their estrogen level rises again, their mood improves. Similar changes take place after the delivery of a baby. During pregnancy, the estrogen level rises about a thousand times over its previous blood level. When the baby is born it plummets, frequently precipitating mood changes and depression.

In a less dramatic but equally valid biological way, your emotions respond to your decreasing estrogen level at menopause. This is a physiological response, though it may be exacerbated, of course, by psychological reactions to this tangible sign of growing older. If you consider menopause a discouraging symbol of approaching age, you'll feel depressed at least temporarily, of course. But your feelings are also influenced by your physical state. If you keep that fact in mind and remember that this too will pass, you can distance yourself from it.

And it will probably pass quite quickly. The emotional component of menopause is an early symptom and almost always fades away in less than a year.

STRICTLY PSYCHOLOGICAL

Whatever feelings are triggered by hormonal changes often become intensified by our feelings about ourselves at this time of our lives. During these same years, much change is often going on in our lives. Many women find themselves alone and struggling. Self-esteem takes a nose dive. Many of us feel as if we were stranded alone in a totally unique dilemma, a stranger in a new land. Few of us in this youth-oriented society can be expected to arrive at midlife, lose our major symbol of youth—our ability to make babies—and have no feelings at all about it. For almost everyone, menopause has its depressing aspects.

This is frequently a time for an identity crisis, a time to assess our accomplishments and abilities and to find them lacking. For most of us, the arrival of menopause seems to focus attention on the negative aspects of our lives, the things we haven't done or been, the opportunities we've missed.

But when you stop to think about it objectively, you will see that menopause need not mean a loss of anything but menstrual periods and concern about getting pregnant. You'll recognize that you can be just as feminine, interesting, and sexually able as you ever were, if not more so. As many women learn more about their bodies at this time and refuse to accept the values and standards imposed upon them by the social mythology about menopause and middle age, they discover that this is but one more chance to take stock of themselves and their lives.

More women are working and developing interests outside their homes and families today than ever before in history. Involved women don't have to find new roles for themselves, new attitudes, and new dependencies when their family situations change—they've already got them. Women are also acquiring greater freedom; they no longer allow themselves to be considered mere appendages to men and children. Just like men, women have a right to be assertive, expressive, sexual, and influential, whatever their age or stage.

If you use this time as an opportunity for reassessment, midlife will give you a new chance at life.

OTHER INTERESTING HAPPENINGS

Menopause is also the time for other bodily changes that may make you wonder what's going on. These changes may not be due totally to low levels of estrogen, but because they tend to start occurring around the time of menopause, it's thought that there is some correlation between them. Here's what we know about them at this writing.

Gaining weight

Most women have a tendency to gain weight after menopause, whether or not they take estrogen. Probably the added pounds can be blamed on a metabolic change because it is obvious that, after about 40, our dietary needs are quite different from what they were in earlier years. Even on the same diet, with the same amount of exercise, you will find it easier to gain weight after menopause. Unfortunately, estrogen therapy won't help. In fact, it may make it even more difficult to stay in shape because it tends to promote water retention.

Changing body shape

After menopause, the actual configuration of the body, the distribution of weight on your bones, begins to change. Hips and breasts tend to lose some of their fat tissue. Waist, shoulders, and upper back often get thicker.

Estrogen replacement therapy doesn't have much effect on weight distribution, though it may help somewhat to keep the weight in its original locations. The most helpful advice we can offer is to keep an eye on your diet and step up your exercise. Cutting down on salt, taking an occasional diuretic or vitamin B6, which is a natural diuretic, will help you fight water retention.

A collection of aches and pains

Other common complaints include backaches, especially in the pelvic area, and muscle pains. One reason for backaches is that one of the jobs estrogen has is to help maintain the protein matrix of the spine and the density of the bones. Its absence may partially explain the aching and feelings of weakness in the back.

The muscle pains probably reflect a reduction in muscular strength as a result of the drop in estrogen, along with a diminished ability to eliminate lactic acid after exercising.

ERT's effect on arthritis

Joint pains, usually caused by osteoarthritis, also tend to occur or become worse around the time of menopause, although nobody knows if there's any connection between them and the new lack of estrogen. We do know, however, that after about two weeks of treatment, ERT often dramatically relieves both muscle and joint pains.

Estrogen may even protect you against developing

rheumatoid arthritis later in your life, according to a new retrospective epidemiological study reported in March 1986 in the *Journal of the American Medical Association*. In research designed to find out whether women who have taken ERT were less likely to get arthritis, a team of epidemiologists at Erasmus University in Rotterdam, The Netherlands, examined the medical histories of 1,000 older women, half already diagnosed with rheumatoid arthritis and the other half with osteoarthritis. Their results showed that those who had taken estrogen replacement earlier in their lives had a dramatically lower statistical incidence (11 percent vs. 36 percent) of rheumatoid (the more serious form of the disease). These findings reinforced earlier research that had indicated that this protective effect seemed to be true for oral contraceptives.

Does this mean you should take estrogen solely to prevent rheumatoid arthritis? My opinion is no, unless you have a strong family history of the potentially crippling disease. However, if you already have arthritis and need ERT's help, you should be delighted to know that taking the hormones will not make your condition worse and, in fact, it may have a beneficial effect.

COPING WITH THE SYMPTOMS

Estrogen replacement therapy will promptly banish all of the temporary symptoms of a changing hormone level. Within a week or two, they'll merely be memories. But if your symptoms aren't too severe or you can't take estrogen because of previous battles with malignancies, there

are some alternative measures that may work well enough
for you. See the next chapter if you want to try them.

THE LONG-TERM MENOPAUSAL EFFECTS

There are three other much more important changes
that are universal among all women who don't take estrogen after menopause. Unlike hot flashes and the other
immediate transient symptoms of menopause that go
away when your body adjusts to the estrogen deficiency,
these are atrophic tissue changes that develop gradually,
always intensify with time, and remain with you forever
unless you take estrogen. They are:

1. Vaginal changes which can make sex extremely uncomfortable or even impossible and which encourage infections.

2. Changes in the urethra which also invite discomfort
and infections.

3. Bone changes, the decreased ability of the bones to
absorb and retain calcium, making them gradually become
brittle and breakable.

Because these three menopausal changes are actual al-
terations of body tissue which can affect the quality of
your life very dramatically, we're going to talk about them
in their own separate chapters.

Most women, if they want to, can manage to live
through the variable transient symptoms of menopause
without medical help because eventually the symptoms
will vanish. But the three universal changes don't fade
away with time. Without estrogen therapy, they get pro-

gressively worse. With it, however, all of them can be reversed or arrested.

HOW THIS BOOK CAN HELP

After a discussion in the next chapter of the alternative treatments for hot flashes and the other vasomotor symptoms, we will take up the three universal changes one by one.

Chapter 7 will concentrate on the effects of menopause on your vagina and therefore your sex life—and what you can do about them.

In Chapter 8, we will focus on the changes in the tissues of the urethra because of your new lack of estrogen, plus vaginal-urethral infections—and what you can do about them.

Chapter 9 is about your bones and your chances of developing osteoporosis—and how you can prevent it.

6

ERT or Not: The Alternative Therapies

IF YOU WAIT long enough, your hot flashes, insomnia, crawly feelings, and other strange vasomotor symptoms will all go away. Time is the cure. If you're one of the lucky ones whom they don't bother very much, just wait them out.

But if you've got symptoms that make you miserable, especially if they last for years, fight back! Refuse to accept them! Take charge of your own life!

Try nonprescription remedies before resorting to any medication, including estrogen/progesterone therapy. All the known nondrug remedies are described in this chapter. But if they don't do the job, remember that replacing the hormones your body no longer manufactures will not endanger your health—no matter what you've heard from friends or relations who recall the scares of the 1970s.

THE NATURAL ROUTE

For vasomotor symptoms that aren't too bothersome, try these natural remedies before turning to ERT or any other medication:

Vitamin E

Vitamin E often does a commendable job of relieving the severity and frequency of flashes and other vasomotor symptoms, and lots of my patients have good luck with it. Start with 400 units twice a day (800 total). If that doesn't work, double the dose for a daily total of 1600 units.

Nobody really knows exactly how vitamin E works because, unlike the other vitamins, it is not a product of the human body. But it produces remarkable results for many women whose symptoms aren't overwhelming.

If you prefer to get your E from your diet—though it is virtually impossible to get as much as you need for this purpose—keep in mind these good sources of the vitamin: wheat germ, wheat germ oil, safflower oil, whole-grain breads and cereals, peanuts, walnuts, filberts, and almonds.

Vitamins B and C

There has also been testimony, though no specific studies to back it up yet, that vitamins B and C can help cool out menopausal symptoms. Try increasing your intakes of both B complex and C. They certainly won't hurt you if you don't overdo them and they may do you some good. Start with one B-50 tablet and 500 mg of C a day and see if you get some relief.

Ginseng

Ginseng, a root that's been used for centuries as a folk medicine to relieve flashes and other "women's troubles," happens to be a potent source of plant estrogen.

If you take it for hot flashes and other vasomotor symptoms, you are now taking estrogen replacement therapy! Ginseng may be a "natural" estrogen, but it is still estrogen and has the same effects on your body as taking the hormone in pills, patches, or creams. Furthermore, this way you are getting it unopposed by progesterone, and so you may build up excessive amounts of uterine lining and develop hyperplasia if you use it continually. Because you can't tell how much estrogen you are getting with ginseng, you'll never know if you are overdosing. This can be dangerous.

So, if you're going to sip ginseng tea to relieve symptoms, do it sparingly, always keeping in mind that you are actually taking estrogen without the protection of progesterone.

Garlic and herbs

There are many herbs—for example, chamomile, catnip, hops, and passion flower—that women who are into natural remedies swear help them with symptoms. Because they have not yet been the subjects of controlled studies, it's impossible to evaluate them objectively. Taken *in moderation*, however, they won't be harmful and they may work for you.

Remember that it is possible—and common—to overdose on herbs. If you do, you may get some unexpected and unwelcome reactions. Some can cause allergic reactions while others can be toxic and hazardous when consumed in large quantities.

Even garlic has been recommended by natural nutritionists and garlic perles are sold in many health-food shops. Certainly, though this possibility has not been scientifically evaluated and seems an unpleasant way to deal with the situation, you will come out way ahead if it helps.

Watch your diet

Nutrition plays an important role in estrogen production, so it's important to be sure your diet is well balanced and adequate. Vegetarians and others who exist on extremely low-protein diets often have such decreased hormone production that they fail to ovulate or to have menstrual periods and end up consulting endocrinologists like me.

So do women who exist for a good portion of their lives on subnormal numbers of calories. Take my word for it, it is *impossible* to get adequate nutrition on less than about

1200 calories a day. Low-calorie diets are unhealthy if you stay on them longer than a week or two. So are high-protein diets, whose devotees include many persistent weight watchers. Besides, they contribute to the risk of developing osteoporosis.

To maintain your hormone output at its optimum before and after menopause, be sure to include all the elements of good nutrition. If you are determined to keep your weight down, choose your menus for health as well as weight loss and avoid extreme low-calorie diets for more than a week at a time.

Cooling off

Do whatever you can to cool off when flashes or heat overtake you. Have a cold drink or a cool shower. They'll help you feel better for the moment. So will air conditioning, layered clothes that you can peel off, cool weather, low humidity, sufficient rest, peace, and serenity. Try them.

Does acupuncture help?

Some women have reported that acupuncture can help relieve the severity and frequency of flashes and other vasomotor symptoms. However, there are no scientific studies that verify this, according to Dr. Fredi Kronenberg of Columbia-Presbyterian Medical Center in New York, who plans to research acupuncture, along with biofeedback and vitamin E, to determine their real effects on menopausal symptoms.

MEDICAL ALTERNATIVES TO ERT

There is nothing that can relieve symptoms as well as estrogen. It works for 98 percent of its users—and it works fast. Within a week to 10 days on a minimal dose, flashes and other vasomotor phenomena are events of the past.

But for symptoms that aren't too severe, you may be able to manage with other treatments. Sometimes they do the job well enough to get you by and are often recommended for women who must avoid estrogen. Here are the alternative medical remedies known today:

Progesterone, the second most important female hormone, may be prescribed alone, without estrogen, to help decrease the frequency and severity of flashes and the other transient vasomotor events. Although it is nowhere near as effective as estrogen, 2.5 mg of oral progesterone a day can sometimes be a helpful alternative when nothing else works.

A long-acting progesterone does work exceptionally well just as it does for symptoms during the perimenopause (page 47), but it has not yet been approved for this purpose by the FDA. This is Depo-Provera, which, injected intramuscularly in doses of 150 mg every three months, usually banishes the symptoms. If your doctor must administer it for a valid FDA-approved use, your troubles are over.

Tranquilizers, especially those like Valium which suppress hypothalamic function, are another medical method for diminishing symptoms. Though they shouldn't be used for long periods of time because they are habit-forming and your body tends to build up a tolerance to them, they sometimes work well. So do *sedatives* which accomplish the goal by decreasing autonomic nervous system irritability. But use them cautiously and only temporarily because they are addictive and potentially dangerous.

Clonidine (or Catapres), a drug normally used for hypertension, sometimes provides some relief from flashes. If you can't take estrogen, this is probably your next best choice after progesterone.

Bellergal is an antispasmodic drug that occasionally diminishes hot flashes, but it is not usually recommended because of its possible side effects. It should be among your last options if estrogen is ruled out for you.

GETTING A GOOD NIGHT'S SLEEP

All the transient and variable menopausal symptoms, including insomnia, usually vanish within a few days after starting estrogen therapy.

But if your symptoms don't seem severe enough to warrant hormone treatment, or you don't choose to go that route, there are other ways to go. The usual remedies well known to insomniacs apply. It's important to remember that your problems with sleep are temporary, probably won't occur every night, and will improve with time.

The over-the-counter sleep medications, usually mild antihistamines, have some sleep-inducing properties and may help you if you use them only occasionally. But try to stay away from prescription sleep inducers because they have a dangerous overdose potential and can become addictive. Besides, they reduce the REM stage of sleep and lose their effectiveness after a while.

Tranquilizers are often prescribed for menopausal insomnia and can be helpful, especially if they are the kind, like Valium, that have a soothing effect on hypothalamic activity. Never use them continually. They can be habit-forming and the body will build up a tolerance to them.

Again, it is best to try the natural remedies before resorting to medications. One is warm milk, which contains tryptophan, an amino acid that acts as a sedative. So do certain other foods such as tuna fish. A tuna fish sandwich and a glass of warm milk could be all you need to put you to sleep for the night! Tryptophan is also available in tablet form if you'd rather ingest it that way and in bigger doses.

Other natural sleep inducers that work for many people include wine (a small amount only, or it may have the opposite effect in the middle of the night), warm (not hot) baths, exercise a few hours before bedtime, ginseng and herbal teas, vitamin B complex, calcium, and vitamin C. Check them out. Remember the precaution about ginseng —you are taking estrogen when you use it.

All the experts on insomnia agree that you probably do get sufficient sleep even with your waking episodes, and the less you worry about it the better. Just remember that the remedy that always works is time. When your body becomes adjusted to its new hormone levels, you'll sleep again.

COPING WITH MOOD SWINGS

Time is once again your best friend. Keep in mind that your physiologically induced mood swings will level out eventually. An early menopausal symptom, they rarely last more than a year. If you decide to start estrogen therapy, they'll improve in a week or so.

Meantime, you may want to join the many women who use nutritional means of achieving better emotional equilibrium. Though there has been no scientific verification of its effectiveness, many people think that taking vitamin B complex—the "antistress vitamin"—is helpful. Though you can get this vitamin in foods such as liver and whole grains, you can also take it in tablet form. Try taking a B complex-50 or -100 capsule every day.

Calcium is also recommended by natural nutritionists for emotional stress, and vitamin C has its supporters who extol it for its calming effect. So does vitamin E, as well as all the soothing herbal teas. If these natural remedies work for you, they may help you avoid drugs.

Obviously, if your emotional state is chiefly due to your changing hormone level, then estrogen replacement can provide dramatic relief. If estrogen works for you—it need be only a temporary measure—you can avoid other more powerful drugs. If it isn't contraindicated in your individual case, try it before you get into tranquilizers or antidepressants.

The hypothalamic-suppressing tranquilizers like Valium are frequently recommended for emotional stress at menopause. They have a sedative and muscle-relaxing effect and can help you sleep, too. Antidepressants are also frequently prescribed and can work wonders for the blues, whatever their source. Get help when you need it!

7

SUPER SEX FOREVER

TAKING ESTROGEN doesn't mean you are guaranteed a great sex life or that all your fantasies will come true. But without it, you may soon have no sex life at all! Estrogen is responsible for maintaining the size, shape, and flexibility of your vagina, as well as the thickness and lubrication of its lining. When you don't produce much of it anymore, certain physical changes take place that can make sex become uncomfortable, downright painful, or even totally impossible.

Astonishingly few women know these facts

of life about sex after estrogen. When their difficulties begin, they are often too embarrassed to talk about them even to their doctors. Most women wait until sex has become miserable before looking for help, or even finding out that help is out there, and a good percentage simply assume their sex lives are over. But spread the word. This is one problem that is easily and rapidly resolved with ERT and has become the primary reason why women start taking it on a long-term basis.

Estrogen restores vaginal tissues to a more youthful state—thicker, moister, more flexible. For women who are already in deep sexual difficulty, the therapy usually reverses the damage in only a few weeks.

That doesn't mean every woman must have ERT after menopause. Some don't need it, at least for several years. For one thing, there really is truth in the warning, "Use it or lose it." An active sex life helps the sex organs remain in good operating condition. Besides, you may be among those fortunate women who continue to manufacture enough estrogen throughout their lives to keep these tissues functioning for a long time.

However, virtually every woman will eventually have to give up sexual intercourse unless she starts taking estrogen.

HOW LONG WILL IT TAKE?

Although some women can't have comfortable intercourse only four to six months after menopause (especially after a surgical menopause), it usually takes 5 to 10 years from the time you lose your primary estrogen source before the typical vaginal problems become acute.

That's why you are lucky if you have a late menopause —these changes will happen much later in your life. A woman who has menopause at 55, for example, will probably not experience serious difficulties until she is about 65. But if your menopause takes place when you are 35, you will be in sexual trouble at a much earlier age, perhaps 40 or 45—unless you take estrogen.

An active sex live will help to delay these changes for another five or even 10 years.

HORMONES AND YOUR LIBIDO

Passing the milestone of menopause doesn't seem to affect the sexual desires of most women one way or the other. Some women, however, find they are *more* interested now that they're not concerned about getting pregnant and have more free time and fewer consuming responsibilities. Many women experience a real sexual reawakening at this time of their lives and it is not unusual for someone who never before experienced orgasms to begin now. Orgasmic ability is unaffected by diminishing hormones.

Other women find their interest in sex wanes with menopause. One good reason is that the physical changes can certainly take their toll on the joy of sex. But interest diminishes very often, too, because women think they *should* be less active and that sex is appropriate only for the young. Some of them, of course, never cared much for sex anyway and use menopause as a convenient excuse to forget it.

HOW TO HAVE SEX FOREVER

In our society, both men and women have been trained to believe that women lose their sex appeal at middle age. That is a false assumption which more and more women are discovering as they begin to toss aside the myths, enjoy the new sexual freedom, keep themselves looking and feeling good, and start making their own judgments.

The ability to have and enjoy sex lasts for a lifetime. It never stops though many women cease to use it. So, assuming you have a compatible partner or the prospect of one, there is no reason not to help yourself to enjoy sex again. Taking estrogen therapy isn't going to give you cancer and it may pave the way to a super sex life.

THE UNIVERSAL PHYSICAL CHANGES

Every woman who is a few years past menopause and doesn't take estrogen experiences vaginal changes. Unlike the early symptoms like hot flashes which, even without help, diminish and disappear eventually, these changes gradually progress with time. The vaginal tissues become dryer, narrower, less pliable and expandable, and occasionally the vagina even becomes a little shorter. In fact, the entrance to the vagina sometimes narrows so much that it won't allow intercourse at all. The vaginal lining loses its tough protective layer of cornified cells and becomes easily injured and irritated and therefore inordinately susceptible to infections.

If you don't want these changes to affect your sexual

activities, you are going to have to deal with them one way or another.

Don't be afraid to discuss your problems with your gynecologist because *you need help*. Fiftyish women are often reluctant to talk about such subjects and, unfortunately, many doctors are reluctant to bring them up. But force yourself to be frank and open so you can get on with your sex life.

LOSS OF LUBRICATION

A vagina that is dry and unlubricated can definitely be a deterrent to sexual enjoyment. This is the first sign of vaginal change and it usually becomes noticeable very soon after—sometimes even before—menopause. When estrogen no longer stimulates the production of cervical and vaginal mucus, the vagina loses much of the lubrication needed for comfortable intercourse. Women who lose estrogen very slowly and continue to make some for many years don't find dryness much of a problem in the early years after menopause, but most women do. An estimated 25 percent of women, only five years into menopause, suffer from vaginal dryness.

When lack of lubrication remains your only problem, it can easily be overcome with lubricants made for this purpose. See below for details.

THE EASILY IRRITATED VAGINA

Lack of lubrication is the first vaginal problem caused by an estrogen deficit. The second is the thinning of the vaginal lining. Without estrogen stimulation, the lining gradually becomes thinner and less elastic so it is easily inflamed or broken and may even bleed.

An easily irritated and inflamed lining can obviously lead to uncomfortable intercourse and a minimal interest in sex. In fact, when the lining becomes so thin that it is virtually nonexistent, sexual intercourse becomes so painful that it is impossible. **At that point, it's essential to start estrogen therapy (via vaginal cream, skin patch, or pill) unless you are willing to give up intercourse forever.**

In addition to providing a happy home for infectious organisms, the thin dry lining sometimes develops a chronic noninfectious inflammation called atrophic vaginitis. Spotting from this kind of inflammation necessitates D&Cs for thousands of women a year because any bleeding requires investigation.

The thinning occurs because one function of estrogen is to stimulate the creation of a tough outer layer of cells (called cornified cells) that protect the more delicate underlying tissues of the vaginal lining against injury and infection. This thickened epithelium appears at puberty and vanishes with menopause. That's why little girls and old women are especially susceptible to vaginal infection. (See the next chapter for more about infections and what to do about them.)

A sidelight: The same kind of layer of cornified skinlike epithelium that covers the entire vagina is also found in the mouth and nose. This tissue, too, tends to thin out and dry when your estrogen is gone. In fact, a prescription for estrogen cream to be applied to the nose stopped severe nosebleeds in a 66-year-old woman recently after nothing else worked!

Urinary inflammation and infections (see the next chapter) are another problem that occur for the very some reason. The urethra and bladder are located adjacent to the vagina. The urethral cells mirror the changes in the vagina and they too thin out with the loss of estrogen. These thinned vaginal and urethral walls mean the urethra can be easily irritated and injured especially during sexual activity, and so it becomes most susceptible to infectious organisms.

THE CHANGING SHAPE OF THE VAGINA

Without estrogen, the vagina reverts to its prepubertal state in another way too. It becomes shorter and narrower and its walls become less elastic. Added to the loss of lubrication and the thinning of the lining, these changes can definitely affect your attitude toward making love.

HOW AN ACTIVE SEX LIFE HELPS

Sex keeps the vagina more elastic, flexible, and lubricated. According to Masters and Johnson, intercourse at least once or twice a week over a period of years will help keep a woman of any age interested and able. The stimulation helps keep the mucus secretions going, maintains muscle tone, and helps preserve the shape and size of the vagina. That's why sexually active women usually have a few years' leeway, delaying the inevitable changes until later in their lives.

But eventually even they will have the same vaginal

dysfunctions other women have—unless they use estrogen.

SEXUAL VARIATIONS

The usual kind of sexual activity—intercourse—is not the only way to help keep yourself in good operating condition, although it is the best. Any method of achieving orgasm, including masturbation, can be useful, and physicians often recommend keeping the vaginal walls toned and shaped with mechanical aids when estrogen is contraindicated or you have no partner.

If this embarrasses you, remember that attitudes have changed and gynecologists today are seeing many more women than ever for sexual problems. In the old days, women with these physical difficulties caused by an estrogen deficit simply accepted their supposedly inevitable fate and gave up sex or the hope of it. Now they look for help. If you need it, do the same.

HOW TO HELP YOURSELF

Let's save the discussion of estrogen therapy for last, and talk about other ways to fend off sexual suicide.

In the early years after menopause when your only difficulty may be vaginal dryness, you can probably do very well with a lubricant such as Surgilube, K-Y Jelly, Transi-Lube, or Ortho Personal Lubricant to prevent the uncomfortable friction of intercourse. Perhaps you'll prefer vaginal suppositories, such as Lubrin Vaginal Lubricating Inserts or Lubafax.

Never use a product that is not designed for this specific purpose, because it can compound your problems. Most cosmetic creams, for example, contain perfume and alcohol that can irritate tender tissues. Don't use petroleum jelly or baby oil because they may cake and dry, causing irritation or damage, provide a habitat for bacteria, and block the release of your own secretions as well. The lubricant you use should be water-soluble and oil-free. The only exception is vitamin E oil, which doesn't dry or cake and may possibly have a beneficial effect on the vaginal lining when lubricants don't help enough. Sometimes, too, vitamin E oil helps to relieve itching and irritation.

By the way, medications such as antihistamines which are designed to dry nasal membranes also tend to dry vaginal membranes.

VITAMIN THERAPY

Whether vitamin supplements will affect sexual desire or performance is debatable, but vitamin E has been credited with beneficial effects and so have the B vitamins. Of course, it is essential to keep your body in good shape by eating well-balanced meals and getting all the nutrients you need, along with sufficient exercise and rest.

WHAT ESTROGEN THERAPY WILL DO FOR YOUR SEX LIFE

It takes only a minimal amount of estrogen in most cases to prevent or remedy every one of the vaginal changes we've described and make sex comfortable again. You'll see results very quickly, noticing some differences in only about two weeks. There's nothing else known today that will do the same job of rejuvenating these tissues.

The lining will start toughening up, lubrication will increase, the tenderness, itchiness, and soreness will be alleviated. By five or six weeks, you will probably be as good as new, though if you've really let yourself go before seeking treatment, it may take a few months to see real improvement.

The estrogen dose must be individualized because some women require more estrogen than others to produce the same results. Always stay with a low dose, however, and *do not fail to take progesterone* as well if you have a uterus. Every woman's vagina can be restored to mint condition with enough estrogen, but the high doses some women need to accomplish perfect results are too high for safety. If this is the case with you, you may have to accept a compromise. But don't worry—there will always be remarkable improvement and you will be in much better shape than you were before. The criteria for successful treatment with ERT are comfortable sex and no more than one or two bouts of vaginal/urinary infections a year.

I strongly recommend that my patients with uncomfortable vaginal changes start ERT if there is no medical reason why they can't. Estrogen has saved untold marriages and relationships and made others possible.

One of our patients, for example, had taken estrogen for about 10 years, then given it up at 57 because of the cancer scare in the mid-1970s. After her husband died and she had no sexual activity, she came for a consultation because of constant vaginal infections. Estrogen was the only solution for her so she started taking it again, with my assurances that it was now absolutely safe if she used it correctly. She is now 68 and has four lovers!

ARE YOU EVER BEYOND REPAIR?

No matter how long your vagina has been out of commission because of lack of estrogen, it will amost invariably regenerate with estrogen therapy. Even if you've been without estrogen for decades, your tissues will probably be restored to functioning condition after only a few weeks or sometimes months of treatment.

PILLS, PATCHES, AND VAGINAL CREAMS

There are three major kinds of estrogen replacement therapy, and each has its advantages and advocates. We'll describe them here and tell you how they can affect your vaginal tissues and therefore your sex life.

Vaginal Cream

If your only postmenopausal problems are vaginal/urinary, you will probably do very well with a vaginal estrogen cream. The topical estrogens, for which a prescription is needed, are absorbed by the tissues of the vagina, plumping them up, encouraging lubrication, and relieving dryness and itching.

How much and how often you use the cream depends

on your needs. Some women require more than others because they don't absorb it as well. It may take experimenting to find out what's right for you.

Always start with a very low dose, perhaps one gram twice a week. It's actually nonproductive to use too much of the hormone because the vagina will absorb only as much as it needs. In the beginning when your tissues are very dry and uncornified, they will absorb a much greater amount than they will later on when they have improved. It only takes three days to a week before the cornified cells start reappearing in the vaginal lining, forming its tough protective layer, and absorption becomes minimal.

By the way, switch to another brand of hormone cream if the one you are using is too sticky or you have an allergic reaction to it. The major objection women have to the cream is its messiness.

Some women use the cream only temporarily until they are in better shape and then go back to lubricants alone. This regime is quite acceptable, though they will inevitably have to resume the treatment after a few months. The symptoms always return when the therapy is stopped and so this must be a lifetime commitment.

Though women sometimes like to use estrogen cream just before intercourse because it does give some local lubrication, this is not a good idea. Your partner may absorb more than is good for him. Besides, if this is the only time you use it, it doesn't have enough time to do its work.

Yes, vaginal cream is estrogen replacement therapy
Don't fool yourself, thinking that if you use vaginal estrogen cream you are not on estrogen therapy. You are. Some of the estrogen you apply locally to your vagina is ab-

sorbed into your bloodstream just like estrogen that's taken any other way. In fact, topical estrogen preparations went out of favor for a while when a study reported there was tremendous absorption from the vagina into the general circulation, with blood levels rising to about 10 times the normal premenopausal levels.

It turned out, however, that this high absorption occurs only in the first few days. When the missing top layer of the lining is replaced through the action of the hormone, the absorption decreases to a fairly minimal amount. Nevertheless, it *is* estrogen and it *does* affect the rest of your body, just like any other estrogen.

Is vaginal cream safe for everyone? As a short-term measure, it is usually considered safe even for women for whom estrogen has been ruled out for medical reasons. The cream is used briefly and temporarily to relieve the worst symptoms and infections that won't respond to anything else. Most women prefer to take a tiny risk if they can get rid of some decidedly miserable chronic vaginal and urinary problems.

The estrogen will also restore their ability to have sexual relations. When the vaginal walls become extremely thin and rigid—as they inevitably do when there is no circulating estrogen—the lubricants won't work. Once the estrogen has restored the tissues, however, the lubricants will be effective enough until the next round of treatment becomes necessary.

An advantage of the hormone cream over oral estrogen is that it is delivered topically. Because it goes directly into the general circulation without passing through the digestive system and the liver, women who can't take hormones by pill because of side effects can get its benefits. The same is true of estrogen taken by way of the new skin patch.

Do you need progesterone too? Because estrogen in any form can cause a buildup of the endometrium, you and your doctor must be alert to that possibility if you still have possession of your uterus. If you bleed with estrogen cream, even with a low dose, you *must* take progesterone too. This is *essential*. The proliferated lining must be shed regularly or it may cause problems later on. See Chapter 12 for more details.

Even if you don't bleed when you are using the vaginal estrogen cream, you should be sure you are really safe from excess buildup of the lining by taking the "progesterone challenge test" after you have been using vaginal cream for a couple of months. This means you take one course of progesterone—your doctor may prescribe 5 mg for 10 days of the month, or perhaps 10 mg for 7 days— while you continue to use the cream. If you bleed, it shows that the estrogen is causing a buildup of the lining and you should take the progesterone every month. If you don't bleed, great. But be sure to test yourself every few months with progesterone.

Reminder: Any unusual bleeding must *always* be investigated thoroughly by your gynecologist. Never ignore it.

And remember, too, that you should have a gynecological checkup every six months, whether or not you have questions or problems.

Oral or transdermal estrogen therapy

For long-term estrogen therapy, it is best to take your estrogen by pill or transdermal skin patch because the dosage can be controlled and you will know how much of the hormone you are getting. When you use the vaginal cream, it is almost impossible to know just how much of the hormone is being absorbed and circulated throughout the body, perhaps affecting other areas such as the endometrium.

Sometimes, when vaginal problems are very severe the results are best if you start taking estrogen by pill or patch *and, at the same time,* use the topical hormone cream for a few weeks too. This builds up the membranes fast and resolves the problems very quickly.

Another good reason to take your estrogen by pill or patch instead of vaginal cream is to protect your bones from osteoporosis. The cream won't do it. Nor are you likely to get sufficient circulating estrogen to affect your skin or your arteries favorably.

In addition, the progesterone you must take every month with oral or skin-patch estrogen may help to protect you against breast cancer.

AS GOOD AS NEW?

Your goals are comfortable sex with no pain during intercourse and no more than one or two vaginal or urinary infections a year, tops.

If you're not reaching those goals, you may have to raise your estrogen dose. (*Never* exceed 1.25 mg of conjugated estrogen or the equivalent dose per day, except under exceptional circumstances and by the direction of your physician.) An alternative is to use the pills or the patch and add one or two local applications of vaginal cream a month.

THE LAST WORD

It's always best not to take any medication, including estrogen, if you don't need it. But when the inevitable vaginal changes make sex too uncomfortable and infections are rampant, you need it. Don't be afraid. Today ERT is not going to give you cancer if you do it right.

8

No More Infections

AFTER MENOPAUSE, when you run out of your major source of estrogen, you may find that you are plagued with one vaginal or urinary infection after another. We're going to give you some sensible suggestions for preventing them and coping with them, but your only hope for a real change in your uncomfortable situation is estrogen therapy. It works by rejuvenating the estrogen-sensitive tissues. For women who get constant serious urinary infections that endanger the bladder or kidneys, ERT is *essential*.

WHY SO MANY VAGINAL INFECTIONS NOW?

Frequent vaginal infections result from the drying and thinning of the fragile vaginal lining now that estrogen is no longer plentiful. Because the lining is easily injured, inflamed, and irritated, it becomes exceedingly vulnerable to all kinds of infectious organisms.

Contributing to the problem, too, is a change in the vagina's acidity balance. In your reproductive years, the normal pH of the vagina is acidic, though there are slight variations thoughout the menstrual cycle. Most of the harmful bacteria and fungi are discouraged by an acidic environment, while the friendly flora which defend you against infection tend to flourish in it.

Once your estrogen level is low, however, the vagina becomes much more alkaline, providing a climate more inviting to many harmful organisms and less suitable for the helpful varieties. That's why women after menopause often get infection after infection and find, just when they think they're finished with one bout, that they're faced with another.

WHY SO MANY URINARY INFECTIONS NOW?

Urinary inflammations and infections also tend to become ordinary everyday occurrences for several reasons. For starters, the outermost portion of the urethra, located just above the vaginal opening, becomes less flexible and elastic with the loss of estrogen. At the same time, its covering membrane thins out. These changes make it more easily irritated and likely to attract infections.

In addition, because of the thinning of the vaginal walls, the urethra and bladder, which are located very close to the vagina, have less protection. That makes them subject to trauma, especially if you are sexually active. The distance between the vagina and urethra becomes shorter, too, allowing infections to cross over from one to the other.

WHAT TO DO

If you have never-ending infections and irritations, your only hope for a real change is estrogen therapy to restore the tissues to a state that's not so attractive to bacteria and other malevolent organisms. Of course, you'll still get an occasional invasion, just as you did when you were younger, but you won't be in the same constant discomfort.

Vaginal estrogen cream applied locally may be all that's required. (Keep in mind that vaginal cream is ERT just like pills or patches, and that some of the estrogen passes through into the bloodstream.) The cream helps by thickening the tissues, relieving the dryness and inelasticity, and encouraging lubrication. It also encourages a more acidic atmosphere. Even women with medical conditions that contraindicate the use of estrogen can usually use the cream safely for short lengths of time.

Oral or transdermal estrogen will have an even more dramatic effect on both the vagina and urethra because more of the hormone will be absorbed and circulated throughout the body.

Normally, only a minimal dose does a good job of banishing recurring infections, though every woman has different requirements. If, even on ERT, you tend to get more than one infection a year, your dose may need to be increased slightly. Or you may need vaginal cream now and then *in addition to* your other estrogen. Don't make these decisions yourself—always consult with your doctor. See Chapter 12 for more details.

Never ignore infections because, while they are sometimes self-limiting, they usually get worse without treatment and therefore harder to eliminate. Make sure your doctor makes the appropriate tests to determine which infection you have before you get a prescription for an antibiotic or other medication. That means that most of the time you must go to the office to have cultures taken. Never use a drug left over from another infection without instruction from the doctor because it may not be appropriate now and will cost you time.

Remember to ask if your sexual partner should be medicated too, since many infections are passed back and forth between partners.

Sometimes it's impossible for your doctor to find out just what organism is causing a minor infection, making it impossible to prescribe the appropriate medication. Try douching with an over-the-counter iodine preparation (Betadine), which may keep the offending bacteria under control.

BEFORE YOUR DOCTOR'S APPOINTMENT

If you can't get an appointment with your doctor immediately and you are having very uncomfortable symptoms such as heavy discharge, irritation, and itching, you can get some relief in the meantime by taking warm baths, or warm baths with a liberal dose of cornstarch. Or try douching with a vinegar solution (one or two tablespoons of white vinegar in one quart of warm water). Baby powder applied externally may also be soothing.

PREVENTING VAGINITIS

To prevent infection, keep yourself in good physical condition. Your immunity to the bacteria which are always lurking around, awaiting their chance, is diminished when you are run-down, tired, or malnourished. Keep yourself scrupulously clean with daily bathing or localized washing with mild nonperfumed soap and water, and be careful to wipe from front to back after a bowel movement to prevent intestinal bacteria from migrating to the vagina or urethra.

TO DOUCHE OR NOT TO DOUCHE

Keeping clean does not mean douching or spraying. Many commercial douches and "feminine hygiene sprays" are irritating and drying, adding to the possibility of infection. They can also destroy friendly flora which prevent pathogens from multiplying. If you feel compelled to douche, do it no more than once a week with plain warm water.

On the other hand, if you tend to get multiple vaginal infections because of your new alkaline environment, mild vinegar douches can help restore the proper balance. Twice a week should be sufficient. Mix one or two table-spoons of white vinegar in a quart of warm water. Your doctor may also prescribe specific douches for specific in-fections.

An occasional douche with baking soda (one table-spoon to a quart of water) will help soothe the itching of fungal infections before they are cleared up.

More Dos and Don'ts

• Again, because the membranes of the vagina are dryer and thinner after menopause, it will always help to use a lubricant during sexual intercourse. This will reduce the friction and help the tissues to stretch without tearing. There are products designed especially for this purpose. Never use petroleum jelly or cosmetic creams. See pages 90–91.

• Wear cotton underpants, or at least pants with cotton crotches. Synthetic fibers have been blamed for re-current vaginitis because they don't allow air circulation, moisture evaporation, or drainage.

• Don't wear pants to bed. Don't wear pantyhose, tight jeans, or synthetic workout gear too much of the time.

• For the same reason, if you are still having

periods, use sanitary pads instead of tampons. That allows more air to reach the vagina.

• No sharing: Because you can pick up organisms from other people, avoid using someone else's douche equipment, bathing suit, panties, towels and so on. Beware of shared hot tubs—the infectious organisms flourish in the hot water and may choose you as their next victim. The chlorine that protects you in a swimming pool evaporates because of the heat of the hot tub's water. One of my patients, a sexually inactive 72-year-old woman, recently picked up a virulent case of herpes from a hot tub.

• Choose your bed partners carefully. If you're sleeping with a new man you don't know or totally trust, make him use a condom. Do the same if he has other sexual partners besides you—or if you're not sure of his fidelity. Simply tell him you can't afford to get an infection.

• Take antibiotics, and penicillin for any reason, only when necessary and under a doctor's supervision. They can upset the pH balance of the vagina, making it even more alkaline and inviting to hostile organisms. They may also kill off the friendly bacteria such as lactobacilli and leave you a likely candidate for fungal infections. Tetracycline is one of the chief offenders, even if you use it only on your skin.

If you must take antibiotics for a prolonged time, you may also need a medication to control the resulting vaginitis.

• Some detergents and soaps can cause irritation, so check them out if you are constantly having problems. Sometimes just switching brands can be make a tremendous difference.

- Never hang a douche bag higher than a foot or so above your hips and never try to force the solution higher than it wants to go. This can wash organisms from the vagina into the uterus.

- Check out your sugar intake. A diet high in sugar encourages fungal infections.

- It may be hard to believe, but you may find relief from vaginitis in yogurt (or acidophilus milk or acidophilus culture in pill form). Lactobacilli, the friendly bacteria normally present in the healthy vagina helping to fight off the harmful sorts, are also found in most nonsterilized (containing *live* culture) yogurt and acidophilus cultures. Nobody knows how many of the lactobacilli that you eat will find their way to the vagina, but many doctors recommend a few ounces of yogurt a day if you are prone to infections. You may have to search for live-culture yogurt—check the labels.

- Vitamin C also seems to help some women fight vaginal inflammation. And some women swear by the B vitamins for the same purpose, so you might try them as a dietary supplement and see if they help you too.

FENDING OFF URINARY INFECTIONS

Most women have no idea that recurring urinary infections have any connection with menopause and the lack of estrogen, but the same hormone deficiency that affects vaginal tissues also changes urinary tissues, making them much more attractive to infectious organisms. Besides, the closeness of the two areas means that infections will often pass from one to the other.

Urinary infections are not only bothersome—painful, itchy, burning, giving you a relentless urge to urinate— but they can travel up the duct to the bladder or even to the kidneys and become serious business.

Sometimes the burning sensation during urination doesn't come from an infection, but is merely the result of a chronic inflammation of the urethra, the vulva, and perhaps the vagina.

STRESS INCONTINENCE

A very common, and not too pleasant, female problem is stress incontinence. This is involuntary urinating that's triggered by a sneeze, a burst of laughter, a hop or a jump.

Usually this condition begins before menopause and gradually becomes worse afterward. There are several reasons for this, but the most usual one is a loosening of the pelvic muscles and connective tissues which hold the pelvic organs firmly in place, especially if you have had at least a few babies. Then your dearth of estrogen makes the tissues even less elastic and strong. At the same time, the sphincter of the bladder which controls urinary flow may have relaxed.

TIGHTEN UP WITH EXERCISE

It may be possible to strengthen the sphincter and the muscles of the pelvic floor that surround the urethra and vagina. If you can manage it, you may alleviate mild cases of incontinence and, at the same time, tone up the vagina. You can do this with exercise.

Every time you think of it, as many times a day as possible, tighten the muscles as if you were trying very hard to hold back your urine. Tight, hold, relax—at least 25 times each session.

Another way to do it: Every time you urinate, start the flow, then stop before you're finished. Holding back, count slowly to 10. Now finish. At first, it may be hard to get to 10, but keep at it and in a couple of months you will probably notice a big improvement.

Severe cases of incontinence, however, often require corrective surgery.

HOW ERT CAN HELP FIGHT OFF INFECTIONS

There is no treatment more effective for constant postmenopausal urinary infections and chronic inflammation than estrogen and it is essential to take it if you're getting little respite between bouts or if your episodes tend to be serious, endangering your bladder and kidneys.

Estrogen revitalizes the urethra, returns some elasticity to the tissues, and thickens the mucous membranes, all defenses against infection. You can take it orally, transdermally, or in the form of vaginal cream.

Some Sensible Suggestions

Whether or not you take estrogen, you can help yourself ward off urinary infections by heeding these sensible suggestions:

- Again, wash with soap and water at least once a day, using a mild nonperfumed, nonirritating soap.

- Concentrated urine provides an excellent breeding ground for invading organisms, so keep your urine diluted by drinking at least eight glasses of water a day. Drink even more if you already have an infection so that you'll empty your bladder frequently.

- Make a practice of urinating at least several times a day. Don't hold on for hours.

- Don't get constipated. A full rectum may cause a backup of urine in the bladder, perhaps partially blocking it so it doesn't empty out totally each time you urinate, providing a happy home for bacteria.

- Urinate before and immediately after sexual intercourse. Infections are often initiated by sexual activity which irritates the urethra and bladder or introduces bacteria into the area. The bacteria then find the urine in a distended bladder a fine medium in which to grow. Also try to drink a lot of water after intercourse to flush out any invading organisms.

- An acid urinary tract fights off harmful bacteria and other organisms better than an alkaline one, and an attempt to make yours more acid could result in fewer infections. A simple way to do it is to drink cranberry juice throughout the day. This is suggested as a preventive, but it may also help clear up an infection. Cranberry juice is cheap compared to drugs, it tastes good, and its acid content matches that of the premenopausal bladder.

Cranberry juice is excreted into the urine as an acid, stays in the bladder as an acid, and so helps keep the urinary tract sterilized. Drink 8 to 16 ounces spaced out through the day. Cranberry juice is calorie-laden so get the low-calorie variety. It can be too acidic for some people and may tend to upset the stomach—but try it.

•   Large doses of vitamin C may also help prevent urinary infections. This is probably because this vitamin tends, like cranberry juice, to make your urine more acid. Taking vitamin C and the juice together is probably the most effective. Again, this may give you a stomach problem.

•   A drug called Mandelamine is sometimes prescribed for persistent infections. It increases urinary acidity and has some antibiotic activity that may keep the infection under control.

•   Try the yogurt-acidophilus route to increase the friendly lactobacilli normally present in the vagina. Be sure the yogurt contains live culture or it won't do you a bit of good.

9

Super Bones
Forever

- Are you thin, fair-skinned, small-boned?
- Did you have menopause before 40?
- Did your mother or grandmother grow shorter?
- Do you smoke?
- Have you gone on a lot of diets, consumed more than two alcoholic drinks a day, always hated milk?
- Does your family come from the British Isles or northern Europe?

IF YOU ANSWER yes to many of these questions, you are in danger of developing osteoporosis, the brittle-bones disease, and I urge you to seriously consider estrogen replacement therapy—the *only* effective way to stop the bone loss that causes it.

Osteoporosis is a bone condition that develops slowly and silently after menopause. There are no warning signs, except perhaps for mysterious backaches, and you probably won't know you're about to have trouble until you do —usually in the form of a fracture—and by then it's too late to remedy the situation. Osteoporosis is not reversible, so early diagnosis and prevention are extremely important.

WHAT CAUSES OSTEOPOROSIS?

If you are a woman with an estrogen deficit, your bones cannot absorb and retain enough calcium—*no matter how much you consume*—to keep them at full strength, and so they start becoming thinner and thinner. Though their chemical composition and structure remain unchanged, they gradually lose much of their mass, bulk, and density. In the first seven years or so after menopause, if you don't take estrogen, the loss is especially rapid.

YOUR CHANGING BONES

Bones are not an inert substance but living tissue that is constantly changing. The skeleton serves as a reservoir for calcium, storing it and then releasing it when it is required by other parts of the body for life-sustaining functions. Old bone tissue is continually being replaced with new so that the skeleton that's yours today is certainly not the one you'll own a few years from now.

Before menopause, there's usually a good balance between the formation of new bone and the resorption of the old—if your diet includes sufficient calcium. But after menopause, resorption overtakes replacement even if you eat your quota of calcium, and so your bones gradually become thinner and weaker.

Bone mass reaches its peak in density at about the age of 35. That's when you have as much bone as you're ever going to get. After that, bone tissue and strength begin to decline in everyone, man or woman.

But women start out with a flimsier bone structure than men and so can't afford to lose as much bone. Indeed, women are four times as likely to get osteoporosis as men, who start with an average of 30 percent more bone mass. Besides, men don't have menopause. The efficient use of calcium is promoted by the male hormone testosterone, which remains in plentiful supply well into old age. In contrast, women's estrogen loss at menopause leads to an accelerated bone loss for about seven years before the rate slows down.

A woman who lives long enough can end up losing as much as 40 to 45 percent of her bones.

Osteoporosis afflicts up to a third of American women over the age of 60 and leads to 1.3 million fractures a year. It's the reason for all those broken hips, fractured wrists, and dowager's humps among the older female population.

Bone loss can never be fully recovered or replaced. Once the damage is done, it's done. The bone that's gone is gone. Since there's no cure for osteoporosis, if you are a woman who is a likely candidate for serious bone loss, you must prevent it before it begins—or stop it before it progresses any further.

CALCIUM ISN'T ENOUGH

Although women have suffered with osteoporosis since the beginning of history, brittle bones have suddenly become big news. We are now bombarded with advice to get exercise and stuff ourselves with calcium to ward it off.

Exercise and calcium will certainly help, but all the physical activity and calcium tablets in the world won't be enough to protect you if you are a prime candidate for brittle bones. The *only* effective way to prevent or arrest this condition is with estrogen replacement therapy *plus*, of course, adequate calcium and exercise.

If you are a high-risk candidate for osteoporosis, you cannot save your bones without estrogen replacement, which ideally should be started within three years of your last menstrual period and continued for life. That's because, if you quit, bone loss begins anew at its accelerated rate.

DOESN'T CALCIUM HELP?

Of course it does. You require adequate calcium as well as exercise to build strong bones and fill the demands for this vital mineral by other parts of your body. But that's only part of the answer. Estrogen, while it isn't directly responsible for bone strength, controls the absorption of calcium into the bones, just as testosterone does for men, and stimulates the production of calcitonin, a hormone that protects bones. When you no longer make much estrogen, your bones quickly start losing more bulk than they gain—*even* if you are eating your quota of calcium.

The bottom line is this: If you've kept your bones at full strength by eating and exercising properly before menopause and have inherited a sturdy skeleton to start with, a calcium-rich diet and moderate exercise may well be all the protection you need after menopause. You probably have enough bone to last you a lifetime.

But if you haven't, you *must* seriously consider estrogen replacement to stem the unrelenting loss of your bone bulk as you get older.

A DISEASE TO RECKON WITH

It's a good thing that osteoporosis has become a popular subject for the media, because it is serious business. It can even be deadly. It symptomatically affects four million women in the United States and becomes severe in a quarter to a third of all white women over 60. It causes over a million fractures, which lead to tens of thousands of deaths a year. Though men get it too, osteoporosis is considered a woman's disease because it is primarily the direct result of diminishing female hormones, beginning its wily work when estrogen grows scarce.

A SNEEZE CAN DO IT

If osteoporosis becomes severe enough, a person who has it could suffer a broken arm lifting a casserole out of the oven or reaching back to zip up her dress. She could break her foot stepping out of bed or a rib because of a sneeze. She could grow noticeably shorter in only a few weeks, develop dowager's hump, have mysterious backaches. Many of the aches and pains of older people result from tiny microfractures and spinal compressions they don't even know they have.

More than 300,000 women a year suffer broken hips because of osteoporosis, with an estimated 30,000 dying of complications and another 100,000 requiring long-term care. One out of every three women fractures a hip before the age of 80. One in five American women over 60 with hip fractures dies of complications, making osteoporosis a leading cause of death in the United States.

Not all women are in serious danger, of course. Those with heavy bones may never be seriously affected because they can lose considerable bone and still have enough to remain strong. But women with light frames have less bone to start with and so they have a smaller safety margin. They need all the help they can get.

WHY CAN'T A WOMAN BE MORE LIKE A MAN?

When it comes to bones, men are far superior to women. They get osteoporosis too, but it develops much later in life for them. Men start out adult life with more massive bones and so they can afford to lose much more bone mass before becoming seriously affected. They also tend to exercise more and eat more calcium-rich foods, especially milk and dairy products, and don't indulge in lose-weight-quick fad diets that are usually high in protein and low in calcium. (If men drink heavily, however, they lose some of their edge. Alcohol hinders the absorption of calcium and often replaces nutritious foods.)

Even more important, the sex hormones—estrogen in women and testosterone in men—have the job of stimulating other hormones that control the absorption of calcium by the bones and inhibit its resorption back into the bloodstream. Men don't lose their testosterone as rapidly and precipitously as women lose estrogen after menopause and so they don't lose bone as fast either.

Because of osteoporosis, the incidence of broken bones rises dramatically in women as they get older, surpassing the incidence in men by far. Though at age 45 the incidence of wrist fractures is roughly equal, it then rapidly rises for women so that, throughout their lifetimes, they suffer 10 times more of these fractures than men do. They have eight times more hip fractures, though at 45 men are six times more likely to break their hips.

About 93 percent of all women in the United States who do not take estrogen will have a fracture of the hip, forearm, pelvis, or spine by the age of 85. The risk for men at that age is just a third of that.

WHO GETS IT?

Everybody gets osteoporosis. It's normal and universal to lose bone as you get older. But severe cases are not normal. It's been estimated that 25 to 35 percent of all women will get it severely enough to cause them real trouble.

--------- **The Demographics of Osteoporosis** ---------

• Osteoporosis is found least often in blacks and most often in whites and Asians. Blacks have been blessed with denser, heavier bones.

• White women of northern European heritage are more likely to develop it than women whose families originated in the southern regions of Europe. A study in Israel found, for example, that the hip fracture rate among Sephardic Jews was only about 60 percent that of European Ashkenazi Jews. As a generalization, it is true that the darker your skin, the lower your chances of developing symptomatic osteoporosis.

• There's more osteoporosis among women living in temperate climates than in the tropics, with Rochester, Minnesota, reporting the highest incidence of hip fractures in the world.

• Accelerated bone loss starts at menopause, no matter what age you have it. That's why women who lose their ovarian function early—say, at 35 rather than 50—are at special risk for major bone loss, especially if they also fit into additional risk categories. Their 15 extra years without estrogen give them more time to develop osteoporosis, and many of them start showing signs of it before they are even out of their 50s.

• Worse than that, women who have very early menopause because their ovaries have been surgically removed are even more likely to have problems a few years down the road because of the abrupt cutoff of estrogen at a young age.

——————— **High-Risk Checklist: Check Yourself Out** ———————

Add up the points for each factor on this list that applies to you. If they total over 6, you should consider yourself at high risk for osteoporosis and take immediate measures to prevent it.

Menopause before 40	3
Family history of osteoporosis	3
Family origin in British Isles, northern Europe, China, or Japan	3
Heavy cigarette smoking (½ pack or more per day)	3
Loss of height, especially in upper body	3
Fracture with no known cause	3
Hyperparathyroid disease	3
Uremia	3
Increased cortisone production or previous long-term cortisone ingestion	3
Vitamin D deficiency state	3
Very fair skin	3
Small bones	3
Consumption of more than 5 ounces of alcohol per day or known liver disease	3
Diet low in calcium	3
Lactase deficiency	3
Malabsorption problem	2

Hyperthyroidism	2
Underweight	1
Sedentary life-style	1
Previous high-protein, low-carbohydrate diet for more than 1 year in adulthood	1

If you are rated at high risk, then you should give serious consideration to estrogen replacement therapy starting immediately after menopause. The *minimum* dosage for prevention of osteoporosis is 0.625 mg of conjugated estrogen a day (or the equivalent dose of other estrogen).

HOW ERT PROTECTS YOUR BONES

According to many controlled studies and a prestigious advisory panel to the U.S. government's National Institutes of Health, estrogen replacement therapy is the most effective way to prevent osteoporosis. It is probably the only way to prevent it from becoming a serious problem, a fact that was borne out by my own 10-year prospective study at Goldwater Memorial Hospital in New York which showed that women who take ERT after menopause do not lose bone while those not taking it definitely do (see details below).

Though other measures, which we'll describe, can help, they cannot compare to estrogen nor will they prevent the disease in susceptible women.

One important piece of evidence in favor of ERT is a

study made by Dr. Bruce Ettinger of Kaiser Permanente in California which compared the effects of calcium supplements alone to those of estrogen on 83 female volunteers who had had menopause six months to three years earlier. Some of the women were given 0.3 mg of conjugated estrogen a day—plus 1500 mg of calcium. A second group received 0.625 mg—and no calcium. The third group took 1500 mg of calcium a day—and no estrogen.

Ettinger compared baseline measurements with bone densities of the women after one year. Those on minimal estrogen (0.3 mg) plus calcium did not lose bone. The women on 0.625 mg of estrogen without calcium also lost no bone mass. But the women who were given 1500 mg of calcium alone without estrogen lost a significant amount of bone.

HOW TO GET YOUR BONES TESTED

The density of your bones can be tested with sophisticated screening techniques such as CAT scans, the single-photon densitometer, which assesses the density of the forearm bone, or the dual-photon densitometer that measures the vertebrae and femur. These are expensive and complicated tests and the equipment is usually available only in large medical centers. They are considered necessary only if you are a high-risk candidate for osteoporosis or have already shown some evidence of it.

A simpler test which can give clues to the presence of osteoporosis is the analysis of a 24-hour urine sample for the ratio between calcium and a substance called creatinine. Because creatinine remains constant in the urine, any change over 0.4 in the ratio indicates high calcium excretion from the kidneys and therefore high bone loss.

Another newly developed test also involves creatinine: This one checks the ratio of calcium with an excreted substance called hydroxyproline. Any amount of hydroxyproline over 0.17 signifies bone loss.

Lost height is a good rough indication of osteoporosis that is already doing its dirty work. The body is measured from the crown of the head to the pubic bone, then from the pubic bone to the base of the heel. The measurements in normal people are almost always exactly the same for both halves of the body. If, however, the upper body is an inch or more shorter than the lower half, you probably have vertebral compression from osteoporosis.

A new test for bone density has recently been developed by the National Aeronautics and Space Administration because astronauts suffer major bone loss during long space flights. Called a bone stiffness analyzer, it uses a probe placed on the forearm or leg bone and an electric current that causes the bone to vibrate. The bone's displacement is then measured. This is a harmless test that takes less than a minute and will probably become a widely used method of detecting early osteoporosis because it shows bone change at a much earlier stage than X rays can.

WHAT ERT DOES FOR YOUR BONES

Estrogen replacement in minimum low doses of 0.625 mg (or equivalent) a day will *prevent* bone loss before it begins, even among high-risk women, if it is started immediately after menopause. It will *stop* osteoporosis from progressing any further, whenever you start it.

WHERE'S THE EVIDENCE?

Many studies have shown that the incidence of spine and hip fractures is reduced among women on ERT, and that bone loss is stopped or prevented. Our own 10-year study, reported in *Obstetrics and Gynecology* in 1976, was the first among the studies that are usually cited as decisive evidence for these conclusions.

In our pioneer research, 168 women, all of them long-term hospital patients, were divided into matched pairs. They were matched by age, physical condition, initial diagnosis, and medication. One of each pair was given daily estrogen/progesterone for a period of 10 years, while the other received placebo tablets identical in appearance. Neither the women nor the researchers knew who received which medication until the study was completed. (Calcium supplements were not included.)

Before the therapy began, each woman was thoroughly examined and tested, and bone-density measurements made. About 40 percent of the women already had discernible signs of osteoporosis, a higher percentage than among the normal population because many of these hospitalized women were confined to wheelchairs or beds and had limited physical activity.

Of the 84 pairs of women, 51 remained in the study at the end of the research when their bones were again measured and analyzed.

The results were highly significant. The women who

began ERT within three years of menopause actually increased their bone mass. Among the women who started taking ERT three years or more after their last menstrual periods and had already lost bone, the condition was stopped in its tracks with no additional loss.

All the women on placebos instead of estrogen, however, showed significant bone loss over 10 years.

Among other well-controlled clinical studies of the relationship of estrogen replacement to bone loss was an important nine-year, double-blind study in Scotland, by Dr. Robert Lindsay and colleagues. The results showed that "a significant reduction in height" occurred among the women who were *not* given estrogen. Conversely, the women on ERT did not get shorter.

Another study led by Dr. Lindsay in the United States concluded that a daily dose of at least 0.625 mg of conjugated estrogen or the equivalent, considered a low dose, is needed to prevent bone loss.

In 1983, the Council on Scientific Affairs of the American Medical Association published a statement concluding that estrogen effectively prevents osteoporosis. And in 1984, the advisory panel to the U.S. government's National Institutes of Health gave a strong endorsement to estrogen for this purpose. The FDA added its approval in 1986.

DO ALL WOMEN NEED ERT?

Of course not. If you've got good strong bones, are not considered at high risk, and have no other serious problems because of estrogen deficiency, you don't need it. It is always best not to take medications you don't need.

However, the preservation of bone structure is one of the most potent arguments in favor of long-term ERT.

DOES MENOPAUSE AFFECT YOUR TEETH?

A study published in the *Archives of Internal Medicine* in 1983 by Harry W. Daniell, M.D., found there is a correlation between tooth loss from periodontal disease and osteoporosis. Tooth loss among white women, he states, is substantially greater after midlife than among men of similar age. According to Daniell, his findings "strongly suggest that middle-aged women may be more likely to retain their teeth if they avoid smoking and undertake a program effective in preventing progression of osteoporosis."

CALCIUM

Do you get enough?

Most women do not consume sufficient calcium at any time during their lives. One study made at the Medical College of Georgia found that the average American female adolescent gets only 700 mg a day in her diet, and older women usually take in less than 500 mg. The National Institutes of Health figures the average woman gets just about half the recommended daily allowance of 1000

mg for premenopausal women and less than that of the
1500 mg dose recommended for those past menopause.

Why you need sufficient calcium

Do you get enough calcium in your diet? Have you
stopped drinking milk under the misconception that you
don't need it after you've grown up? Do you worry so
much about cholesterol and getting fat that you've eliminated some of the foods that are best for you? If you are a
typical American woman, it is most unlikely that you get
your optimum calcium every day, especially since you're
probably perennially on a diet. It's *impossible* to get enough
of the mineral from food when you eat very few calories.

The essential fact to remember is that, when there's
not enough calcium available from the food you eat, your
body will take what it needs right out of your bones.
Young women should eat sufficient calcium because it's
vital to start out with the maximum allotment of bone.
Older women should be especially conscious of calcium
consumption because, without enough of the mineral on
hand to supply vital body functions, your bones will be
plundered to provide it. Besides, your absorption is not
what it once was.

For this reason, *calcium supplements are essential for most
women.* Before menopause, you need them if you're not
going to drink four glasses of whole or skim milk (skim
milk retains all the calcium of whole milk) or their equivalent a day. The same applies if you are on ERT after menopause. But if you don't take estrogen, you need
supplemental calcium unless you consume at least *five*
glasses of milk or their equivalent daily.

——————— How Much Calcium Do You Need? ———————

• Before menopause, you should have a mini-mum of 1000 mg of calcium per day in food and/or supple-ments.

• If you have had menopause *and* take estrogen, you also require at least 1000 mg.

• If you have had menopause and do *not* take es-trogen, you need a minimum of 1500 mg a day.

_____

Some Asides to Remember

• Calcium is best absorbed if it's consumed throughout the day, rather than all at once. So divide your daily dose into halves or thirds and space it out, or take time-release capsules. It is also absorbed better if you take it with meals.

• Antacids which are aluminum derivatives (al-hydroxides) take calcium from the body. Check the labels for these ingredients if you habitually take them for heart-burn, hiatus hernia, and so on, and don't use them as a calcium source. Switch to another kind.

• If you eat a very high-fiber diet, be sure to com-pensate with extra calcium especially if you are at high risk for osteoporosis. A large consumption of fiber, though it is beneficial in many ways, causes your intestines to ab-sorb less of everything, including calcium, because the food passes through your body so rapidly.

• Don't rely on leafy green vegetables for your major source of calcium. We will explain why below.

Money in the bank?

There's a theory that, if you overdose on calcium during your years of growth and young adulthood, you'll build heavier denser bones that will serve as "money in the bank" for the future. But your bones can only get as thick and dense as your genes have preordained them to become. While you certainly need enough calcium to build them to their optimum size and strength, they can only reach their own genetic potential.

In other words, *your bones can't get any thicker or heavier than your genes have programmed them to be at about age 35.* Once you have reached your threshold for calcium, more is useless. It may even be harmful if your kidney function is less than optimal or you have a tendency toward kidney stones. Overdosing is not recommended.

Good food sources of calcium

We should all eat foods rich in calcium, especially after menopause. If you don't like your milk straight, eat cheese, yogurt, or any other milk products instead but be sure to eat enough of it. Check the calcium content of some of the top calcium food sources in the table below, add up what you typically eat in a day, and make sure you get at least 1500 mg if you don't take estrogen and 1000 if you do. If you can't manage to get that much in your diet, then you'll need calcium supplements. Include sardines or other soft-boned fish such as canned salmon and leafy green vegetables such as collards, kale, and turnip greens.

Caution: Many leafy greens, including spinach, beet

greens, and Swiss chard, are actually calcium *blockers*. They contain oxalic acid which inhibits the body's absorption of calcium. So, even though they are chock-full of this valuable mineral, you won't get the entire benefit of it and, in fact, when you eat them with milk or other calcium sources, you may be blocked from getting much of the benefit of *their* calcium as well.

Although many other foods, from sesame seeds to oysters, contain calcium, let's face it: **It's virtually impossible to get your daily allotment of 1000 to 1500 mg in your diet without consuming considerable amounts of milk or milk products.** If you don't drink enough milk or eat enough dairy products, you need calcium supplements to bring the numbers up. Your body couldn't care less where the mineral comes from.

——————— **Some High-Calcium Food Sources** ———————

FOOD	PORTION	CALCIUM
Milk, whole	1 cup	291 mg
Milk, skim	1 cup	302 mg
Yogurt, whole milk	1 cup	274 mg
Yogurt, skim milk (with added nonfat milk solids)	1 cup	452 mg
Swiss cheese	1 oz	272 mg
Sardines, canned	3 oz	371 mg
Salmon, canned	3 oz	167 mg
Mackerel, canned	3 oz	205 mg
Oysters	1 cup	226 mg

————— **Some High-Calcium Food Sources,** *cont.* —————

FOOD	PORTION	CALCIUM
Broccoli, chopped, cooked	1 cup	180 mg
Turnip greens, chopped, cooked	1 cup	198 mg
Collard greens, chopped, cooked	1 cup	148 mg

Choosing a calcium supplement

When you come upon a store counter stacked with bottles of calcium supplements, which should you choose? According to the Center for Science in the Public Interest, your body absorbs all types of calcium equally well. The major difference is how much elemental calcium you are getting in each pill. With less concentrated sources, you have to take more pills to end up with the same amount of calcium.

Many of these supplements are made from calcium carbonate, which is easily absorbed, supplies a lot of calcium per tablet, and is usually inexpensive. However, it sometimes causes excessive gassiness or constipation. Calcium phosphate supplements provide the same amount of calcium per tablet but without the gas-producing side effect. Calcium lactate contains less than half the amount of available calcium per tablet, and calcium gluconate contains about a quarter of the amount supplied by the same size tablet of calcium carbonate or calcium phosphate. Calcium citrate is probably the least likely to result in kidney stones.

Many women like to take oyster-shell calcium because it is natural, like sardines. It is a perfectly good source of calcium carbonate. So are some antacids. However, five or six tablets a day are needed to reach the U.S. government's RDA. Remember to avoid using the antacids that are aluminum derivatives (alhydroxides), because they *remove* calcium from the body.

Taking bonemeal or dolomite as a source of calcium is not a clever idea. While they contain calcium, they also may be contaminated with lead or other toxic metals. Besides, they may be poorly absorbed by the body.

WHAT ABOUT VITAMIN D?

Without vitamin D, the body can't absorb calcium, but most people get plenty of D from sunlight and diet. So unless you're very old, cooped up in the hospital, and eating poorly, don't worry about it. If you take too much of it, it may have the opposite effect from the one you want and actually make you *lose* bone.

If you want to add vitamin D to your regimen, as many women do, take only a minimal amount—250 international units a day is plenty. More than 20,000 international units per day can be toxic. Check out your calcium supplements. If they include vitamin D, add up the total you'll be taking in a day and be sure you aren't getting too much.

You especially don't need vitamin D supplements if you are taking estrogen because it increases the production and absorption of the vitamin (in its activated form of calcitriol) by the body. The estrogen plus sufficient calcium are all that's required.

WILL SODIUM FLUORIDE HELP?

People who live in high-fluoride areas show a greater average bone density than those who reside in low-fluoride areas, because fluoride does seem to encourage the retention of calcium in bones as well as teeth.

A new study from Finland suggests that older people who have been drinking fluoridated water have less fragile bones, resulting in a much lower rate of fractures. According to the study, a small amount of fluoride in the drinking water can lower the number of hip fractures in older women by about a third.

But in spite of the fact that other research indicates that treating seriously osteoporotic women with fluoride also lowers the fracture rate (even though the "bone" it stimulates is not normal bone but a hard collagen-like substance), it has not yet been approved by the FDA. Besides, it can cause a vast array of side effects, including joint and tendon inflammation, anemia, and gastrointestinal disturbances.

WILL CALCITONIN INJECTIONS HELP?

Calcitonin is a body chemical that's needed for the absorption of calcium, but using it as a treatment for osteoporosis is valid only if you have a serious calcitonin deficiency. It must be taken in a daily injection, a difficult regime. Also, if you are lacking that much calcitonin, the most likely reason is your low level of estrogen. Therefore, the best way to increase it is to start ERT.

DOWN WITH LOW-CALORIE HIGH-PROTEIN DIETS!

If you're looking to lose weight in a hurry, a quickie high-protein diet is okay for a week or so, but never longer. It's not healthy. One reason is that it leads to acidosis. Even moderate acidosis increases the excretion of calcium from the kidneys and can cause osteoporosis over a long enough time, making women who persistently follow bizarre diets that don't include the normal balance of foods more likely to develop brittle bones. There is also some evidence that excessive consumption of animal protein blocks calcium absorption and, in fact, vegetarians tend to have denser bones than meat eaters.

ALCOHOL AND YOUR BONES

Alcohol speeds up the loss of bone tissue and the two are dose-related. Big drinkers lose bone at a faster rate than moderate consumers or teetotalers. They tend to eat less nutritiously and, in addition, the alcohol inhibits calcium retention. So excessive bending of the elbow is ill-advised for this reason, among others.

SMOKING AND YOUR BONES

Smoking puts you into one of the highest-risk groups for osteoporosis, partly because it can cause an earlier menopause then you were genetically programmed to have, giving you more years of fast bone loss, and partly for reasons we don't yet understand. Bone loss is about twice as rapid among thin postmenopausal women who are heavy cigarette smokers (at least 10 cigarettes a day for five years or more) as it is among thin postmenopausal nonsmokers. Men who smoke are 2.3 times more likely to get it, too.

If you want to fend off osteoporosis, stop smoking!

CUT DOWN ON SALT

As if you needed it, here's another reason besides aggravating hypertension and water retention to cut back on salt. A new study in The Netherlands found that high intake of salt increases the excretion of calcium, which means less is being retained by the bones.

CAFFEINE AND YOUR BONES

If you drink more than moderate amounts of coffee, tea, or anything else that contains caffeine, you may add to your bone loss. High caffeine consumption causes acidity just as a high-protein diet does.

HOW EXERCISE HELPS YOUR BONES

Bones are like muscles—if you use them, they get stronger and thicker. If you don't use them, they become weaker.

To build and maintain strong bones throughout life, you need exercise, though nobody knows just how much is required to do the job. What we do know is that the activity you choose must provide the mechanical stress of muscles pulling on bone, and must be weight-bearing and antigravitational. The absence of gravity is why astronauts develop osteoporosis.

As far as bones are concerned, the benefits you achieve from exercise are exceedingly specific: They occur only at the specific sites that are actually stressed. For example, runners will get the major benefit in their legs, while tennis players will find that the bones in their dominant arms get thicker.

Bones respond to physical activity at any age, though menopause is the time of our lives when most of us exercise less and sit more; in fact, a lot of women over the age of 50 still think exercise is dangerous for them. The truth is, it isn't dangerous and we need it even more than ever to keep every part of our bodies in optimal shape. Remember, though, that you need adequate calcium too. Exercise alone won't affect bone mass.

Exercise that benefits bones

Almost any kind of vigorous exercise makes you more fit, strengthens your heart and lungs, tones up your muscles, and makes you feel mentally alert. But to build bone, vigorous aerobic exercise isn't enough. Your physical activities must be the kind that stresses the long bones of the body and adds the force of gravity: for example, jogging, brisk walking, bicycling, dancing, and any form of jumping and running. Swimming, great for other reasons, won't do as much for bones because the water cancels out the effects of gravity.

Incorporate an exercise program into your life as a reg-

ular event, at least a half hour four times a week. You'll be
doing your bones a real service.

ERT: THE LASTING EFFECTS

To prevent osteoporosis, estrogen replacement must
be a long-term commitment. As long as you take the hormone, your bones will be preserved. When you stop taking it, the benefits cease and you'll start losing bone again.

You'll still come out ahead, however. That's because
for whatever time you take ERT, you are gaining invaluable time. If, for example, you take estrogen for five years,
then stop, your bones will be five years younger than if
you hadn't taken it at all.

On the other hand, when you quit, the bone loss will
be especially rapid for a few years, just as it would have
been immediately after menopause if you hadn't started
ERT.

Any form of ERT improves the absorption of calcium
by the bones, even vaginal cream to some extent. But for
this purpose, oral estrogen has been proven to be far superior. Preliminary two-year studies have indicated that
the new transdermal patch will give the bones just as
much protection.

NEVER TOO LATE

Whenever you start ERT, it will do its job of arresting
bone loss. I've had patients 80 or 90 years old benefit sig-

nificantly from ERT that was prescribed to stop osteoporosis from advancing further.

ADDING IT ALL UP

The bottom line is that nothing will preserve your bones like estrogen. It's the single most important approach to the prevention and treatment of osteoporosis.

10

Your Skin: Will Estrogen Keep You Young Forever?

No, ESTROGEN is not the fountain of youth and it won't keep you young forever. But it can certainly make a difference in the way you look. Though it won't stop the clock or prevent the skin changes that happen normally with the years, it can affect those processes that are under its own specific control. It will help you look younger, sometimes years younger, than you would have looked without it. **Women on estrogen replacement therapy definitely tend to look more youthful than their years. Their skin stays thicker, moister, oilier, and more flexible. Their muscles remain firmer, their hair stronger.**

Consider this only a delightful fringe benefit of ERT because few specialists in women's health would recommend taking estrogen for this reason alone. After all, hormones are drugs and we still don't know everything there is to know about them. But if you take them for valid medical reasons, your skin will certainly prosper as a result.

THE NATURAL HISTORY OF SKIN

As we get older, there is a normal and gradual breakdown of collagen or connective tissue and the elastic fibers of the skin, the largest and most visible organ of the body. And, at the same time, there's a gradual decrease in thickness and lubrication. The skin becomes dryer. Muscle and fat tissue gradually shrink, while the skin tends to stretch.

Overexposure to the sun, the skin's archenemy, hastens the procedure by leaching out moisture permanently, destroying oil glands, collagen, and elastic fibers in the dermis, the deep layer of the skin, making it lose much of its softness, flexibility, and natural lubrication.

Smoking speeds up the damage, too, by constricting the skin's blood supply and allowing less oxygen to reach the dermal cells. Drastic dieting, quick weight changes, plus years of living in an environment consistently low in humidity also play their parts.

ESTROGEN'S ROLE IN YOUR SKIN

It's important to know how estrogen specifically affects the skin, because it is these effects that can be delayed or even somewhat reversed by taking estrogen supplements, though the hormone can't do anything to moderate the changes that happen simply because we are getting older or inflicting damage on our fragile exteriors.

A British study reported in 1985 that the condition of the skin depends more on the "age of menopause" than on chronological age. In other words, it correlates more closely with how many years you've been without estrogen than with how old you are.

Estrogen is largely responsible for the distribution of subcutaneous fat, the layer of fat just under the epidermis that provides inner support, firmness, and resilience. So when you lose your major supply of this hormone, the delicate balance between estrogen and androgens, the malelike hormones that all females naturally produce, is upset. With less estrogen, the androgens exert more influence throughout your body. In the skin, the subcutaneous fat layer gets thinner at a result, losing much of its natural padding.

Estrogen is responsible, too, for maintaining water in the tissues by stimulating the production of a substance called hyaluronic acid which holds the water. A lack of estrogen lowers the extracellular moisture content of the skin, allowing it to dry out. In addition, without the influence of estrogen, the skin produces less and less oil for lubrication.

The third important effect on your skin after menopause is a measurable decrease in its thickness. Without estrogen, collagen, the connective tissue that keeps the skin thick and firm, gradually becomes depleted, giving the skin more opportunity to wrinkle.

In men, skin thickness declines linearly with age, but in women, there's a sharp decrease in the fifth decade.

Research at King's College Hospital in London found that skin is only half as thick in women nearing 60 who do not take estrogen as it is among those who do.

WE'RE ALL DIFFERENT

Of course, changes in the skin and the degree to which they happen differ for all of us. Some fortunate women inherit wonderful skin that remains firm and smooth in spite of the passing years if they don't grossly abuse it. In general, these are the ones who do not experience a sudden tremendous drop-off of estrogen at menopause and who continue for most of their lives to produce a certain amount of the hormone, mainly now from their adrenals and fat cells.

Women who have a late menopause also have a big advantage over those who lose their estrogen early. Because they have more years of circulating estrogen affecting their skin as well as the rest of their bodies, they frequently have firm smooth skin even if they don't go on ERT and tend to look younger than their peers.

Women with a little extra weight usually look younger after menopause too, not only because they continue making estrogen in their fat tissue, but also because their extra fat plumps up their skin. If you make a survey of your friends and neighbors, you'll find the skinny ones usually look years older than those with a few extra pounds.

WHAT ESTROGEN DOES FOR YOUR SKIN

For optimal effects on your skin, ERT must be started very soon after menopause. That's because, just like the bones, the skin changes most rapidly during the first several years after your major source of female hormones is gone. But whenever you start, you are likely to see some improvement.

Although estrogen can't totally reverse any damage that's already been done by estrogen deficiency and certainly can't change the effects of aging and overexposure to the sun, it can help hold off further changes due to estrogen loss and improve your skin by adding fat, moisture, oil, and collagen.

By increasing local fluid retention, estrogen puffs the skin up to a certain degree and thereby helps to smooth it out. For some women, this makes a dramatic difference in the way they look. The fluid retention, however, lasts only as long as ERT is continued. (Of course, if the water retention also occurs in the ankles or other parts of the body, it may not make you so happy.)

The additional subcutaneous fat stimulated by ERT makes the skin a little tighter, and the increased oil production keeps it from drying out as much as it otherwise would have.

The collagen retention causes it to become progressively thicker. The longer you continue to take estrogen, the thicker your skin will get (up to a point) as more collagen is deposited to build up the layers. If you quit the therapy, your skin will then start losing its thickness again, as well as its moisture, oil, and fat, though you will still come out ahead of the game because you have started off with more tissue than you would have had without it.

WHAT ELSE IS GOING ON?

More sweat: After menopause, you'll find you may perspire a lot more than you ever did before. That's because the androgens, the malelike hormones, are no longer so tightly controlled by estrogen, making your sweat glands work more efficiently.

It's not known if concentrations of melanin or pigmentation—oversized freckles or liver spots—are initiated by the change in female hormone levels. But we assume they are because they do tend to make their first appearances around the time of menopause, showing up mostly on the face, neck, hands, and arms, the areas most exposed to sun over the years.

SAVING YOUR SKIN WITH OR WITHOUT ESTROGEN

Good skin care can make an enormous difference in the way your skin looks and lasts. Whether or not you are on estrogen therapy, there is much you can do to keep your skin looking younger and fresher.

• Stay out of the sun; it is your skin's major enemy and its damage cannot be reversed. When you must be exposed, use a sunscreen and acquire a light tan only gradually. Reapply the sunscreen every hour or so and after washing, swimming, or working up a heavy sweat. Never use oil or cocoa butter or any other kind of grease to encourage tanning because it also encourages burning and damage.

- Try to maintain an environment that is reasonably humid. If you live in a dry climate, a humidifier is a wise investment.
- Use moisturizer faithfully to seal in the water already present. Apply it to skin that's been given an opportunity to absorb water first—immediately after a bath or a wash. Avoid dehydrators; these include alcohol, caffeine, diuretics, dry air, and saunas.
- Drink plenty of water—eight glasses a day is the dermatologists' recommendation.
- Oil up your skin regularly (petroleum jelly, any oil, vegetable shortening, or something fancier will do).
- Skip soap or use superfatted soap for cleansing or, if you prefer, a creamy cleanser for face and neck.
- Get plenty of vigorous exercise. Healthy circulation will improve blood circulation to the skin as well as every other part of the body. Toned muscles will help round out your contours, too.
- If you must diet, lose weight slowly. Quick weight loss can have a devastating effect on your skin at this time in your life.
- Use oil-based cosmetics and avoid perfumed skin products because they are drying.
- Be sure to consume small daily amounts of vitamin C. Research from Duke University Medical Center shows a link between this vitamin and collagen synthesis.

ARE ESTROGEN CREAMS HELPFUL?

Creams containing estrogen, though they may improve your skin, are not recommended simply because the estrogen can affect much more than your outer layer. The hormone is absorbed into the bloodstream just like any other estrogen and has been known to cause vaginal bleeding in women and breast development in men and children. Beware!

AND COLLAGEN CREAMS?

There is no evidence that the collagen (connective tissue) added to "collagen creams" can be absorbed into the skin. If any scientific research has been done on this subject, the medical community is not yet aware of it. The collagen may, however, help the skin retain moisture because it holds water, but then so does any moisturizer.

A COSMETIC DRAWBACK TO ERT

ERT occasionally causes increased pigmentation, a slight darkening of the skin here and there. Sometimes moles get darker and larger and tiny papillomas appear, especially on the neck and chest, just as they frequently do in pregnant women and women on oral contraceptives. Though you may not care for them, they are not harmful.

HOW ESTROGEN AFFECTS YOUR HAIR

One of the jobs of estrogen is to encourage the growth of hair on the head, the pubic area, and under the arms, and to discourage it on the rest of the body. With the advent of menopause, that pattern tends to change. Some women notice that the hair on their heads starts to get thinner, and that the secondary hair—in the armpits and pubic area—becomes straighter and less luxuriant.

At the same time, usually five or more years after menopause, hair may start growing here and there on the face and body where it never grew before and where it certainly is most unwelcome. Adding to the problem, the hairs already there often become darker, thicker, and tougher. All this happens because, once again, the androgens that every woman naturally produces are activated as the estrogen level drops. Estrogen no longer blocks the action of these malelike hormones at the hair follicle receptors and so the hair tends to grow in a more male pattern.

Though estrogen levels don't affect hair color, they do influence texture and oil. The hair on the head usually becomes coarser and always much dryer. Estrogen therapy won't have an enormous effect on the hair on your head, though it may thicken it up a little. But it will have a beneficial effect on the unwanted facial and body hair. When you start ERT, the hair growth in these areas stops, though the hairs already there will remain until their life span is completed or you remove them.

An alternative to ERT is a drug that is not yet approved for this use by the FDA, though it has been approved as a potassium-sparing diuretic. This is spironolactone, marketed as Aldactone, which is a specific receptor blocker for face and body hair and may be helpful in encouraging the growth of hair on the head. Its action as a diuretic is extremely mild and so your doctor may agree to prescribe it in an effort to alter the pattern of your hair growth. A drawback is that you'll probably revert to your former pattern when you stop using the drug.

The only permanent way to remove unwanted hair, by the way, is with electrolysis, which should be done by a reputable and experienced operator recommended by your doctor. The other routes to take are effective but imperfect and temporary. Tweezing works but it does not remove the hair by the root and may encourage infection. Shaving is unaesthetic. Depilatories may be irritating to delicate skin, and waxing, another temporary measure, is uncomfortable and may cause ingrown hairs.

A FINAL WORD

We're not recommending estrogen replacement as a beauty aid. Estrogen is a drug, not a cosmetic, and it should always be treated as one—with caution and respect.

11

Hysterectomies, Oophorectomies, and Instant Menopause

An astonishing number of women are totally confused about what goes on during a hysterectomy. They don't know what's removed during the surgery or how the procedure may affect menopause, their estrogen supply, and their lives. That's why, in this chapter, we're going to answer the questions patients always ask and try to straighten out some common misunderstandings.

WHAT HAPPENS WHEN

When you have a simple *hysterectomy*, your uterus and cervix (or a portion of the cervix) are removed. Your ovaries remain intact. If you haven't had menopause, you will continue to make estrogen from your ovaries and you will not have menopause now. You'll have it whenever you would normally have had it. You won't, however, have any more menstrual periods and you can't get pregnant. And obviously, because you haven't had menopause, you won't get any of its typical symptoms at this time.

When your ovaries are removed in an operation called an *oophorectomy*, you will have *instant menopause* if you are still having periods. From that moment on, you will make no more estrogen (except for the small amounts made in the adrenals and fat tissue) and you will have no more menstrual periods. Obviously, you can't get pregnant either. You will probably have severe menopausal symptoms starting within a day or two of the surgery.

Occasionally, only one ovary is removed. In this case, the above doesn't apply because the remaining ovary will keep on turning out hormones until you have a natural menopause.

Often both a hysterectomy (removal of the uterus) and an oophorectomy (removal of ovaries) are performed together, and most people, doctors included, usually refer to the surgical procedure as a "hysterectomy" even though in this case it's much more than that. This misuse of terms causes a lot of confusion. It's clear that we need a new word that covers this double happening.

It's important to know whether you've had one or both

surgical procedures—in other words, whether you still possess your ovaries. Many women have no idea whether they do or not, and it's always amazing to me how many assume that, of course, "everything" has been removed. The women whose ovaries (or one ovary) are still intact are often mighty surprised years later when their estrogen production tapers off and they start getting menopausal symptoms. A lot of them go to their doctors thinking they have developed some rare disease!

After a hysterectomy, the ovaries do not shrivel, as many women seem to think. They have their own blood supply and continue to function. However, if the uterus is removed at a relatively young age, menopause often arrives earlier than it would have otherwise, sometimes by a number of years. The reason is that some of the blood circulation to the ovaries may have been compromised during the surgery.

Women often wonder if they continue to ovulate after a hysterectomy and, if so, what happens to the eggs. The ovaries do continue to produce eggs every month, though these eggs can't be deposited into a nonexistent uterus for possible fertilization. So they are expelled into the abdominal cavity where they are quickly and harmlessly absorbed.

WHO NEEDS A HYSTERECTOMY?

Most hysterectomies are performed because of large and bothersome fibroids, nonmalignant tumors that can cause heavy bleeding and sometimes, if they become large enough, pressure on the bladder, the ureter, or the rectum.

Sometimes hysterectomies are recommended because of serious infection, severe pain, or other problems. And very rarely a uterus must be removed because of cancer.

Hyperplasia, the building up of too much uterine lining, is another common reason for surgery, performed out of fear the hyperplasia might become malignant. Sometimes it is actually *mistaken* for cancer.

Always get a second opinion or even a third opinion before agreeing to surgery for hyperplasia, however, because in the vast majority of cases the overproliferated lining can be reversed very simply and thoroughly with two or three months of treatment with progesterone. The hormone, taken by pill, inhibits the growth of the lining. Almost invariably, it quickly restores the lining to a normal healthy state, with no surgery required.

WHEN OVARIES ARE REMOVED

If your ovaries are removed in an oophorectomy (or rendered nonfunctioning because of other damage, such as radiation) before you have had menopause, you will have instant and absolute menopause. And you will have instant symptoms, symptoms that are probably much more severe and long-lasting than they would have been after a natural menopause.

That's because of the very sudden drop in hormone levels. Women who have surgical menopause usually have the most uncomfortable symptoms of all, starting a day or two after the surgery. In fact, the younger you are at the time of the surgery, the worse the symptoms are likely to be and the longer they will tend to last.

Most premenopausal women who have an oophorectomy are promptly given estrogen replacement therapy for at least six or eight weeks and so have none of the usual discomforts until and unless they decide to give up the treatment. Ovarian cancer, by the way, does not necessarily rule out the use of ERT as do uterine cancer or estrogen-dependent breast cancer (see Chapter 12).

The other major disadvantage of losing your ovaries before they are ready to quit making estrogen is that you now have extra years without the hormone's benefits and so more time to develop the consequences of estrogen deficiency—osteoporosis and urogenital problems, as well as a significantly higher risk of heart disease. If you take estrogen, however, you can avoid all of them.

If you've already had menopause before you have your ovaries removed, you probably won't have any of the transient menopausal symptoms again, though occasionally they'll make a brief appearance. If that happens, it is because you were still making a minimal amount of estrogen from your ovaries, though not enough to stimulate ovulation and menstrual periods.

KNOCKING OUT THE OVARIES NONSURGICALLY

Sometimes the ovaries are deliberately destroyed by radiation, as an alternative to surgery. And sometimes the destruction occurs as a side effect of radiation treatments of the pelvis or abdomen. Chemotherapy, too, can render the ovaries nonfunctional. When they are knocked out quickly for any reason, menopause is instant and the symptoms are usually sudden and severe if you don't promptly start hormone supplements.

IS ESTROGEN REPLACEMENT NECESSARY?

ERT isn't necessary but it certainly makes life a lot easier because of the intense symptoms you are likely to have without it. That's why few women fail to take it and few doctors refuse to prescribe it. With the current methods of administering estrogen replacement therapy, there is nobody for whom it's not safe except those who have had uterine cancer or estrogen-dependent breast cancer.

ERT is usually continued for about five years after the surgery, which is considered short-term, or until you wish to end it. Be sure to stop gradually if you decide to quit, or you may find yourself having to cope with the same symptoms all over again.

Obviously, if you no longer have a uterus, you don't have to take progesterone because you can't possibly get endometrial cancer. Nevertheless, it is an excellent idea to take it anyway for its probable protection against breast cancer.

If you cannot take estrogen, then you must cope with the withdrawal symptoms, such as hot flashes, in alternative ways. See Chapter 6.

WHY YOU SHOULD KNOW IF YOU HAVE OVARIES

If you have had an early hysterectomy but have kept your ovaries, you can expect to have menopause around the time when you would normally have had it. But many women can't believe it when they start having hot flashes years after their surgery. "How is that possible when I've had a hysterectomy?"

Aside from avoiding a big surprise a few years down the road, you should know whether or not you have ovaries for another reason: When you go to a new doctor, you should be able to give a complete medical history so the doctor can be alert for problems such as cysts or enlargement or infection of the ovaries.

If you don't know your internal status, ask your present or former physician to check the records or request that the hospital look into its surgical reports. Failing that, your new doctor can find out if you are approaching menopause by measuring your FSH level. It will be elevated if the ovaries are gone or nonfunctioning, or if you have had menopause.

SHOULD YOUR OVARIES BE REMOVED TOO?

Sometimes ovaries are removed surgically because they are diseased or nonfunctioning or because a malignant tumor, usually in the breast, has been judged to be estrogen-dependent.

But most often ovaries come out along with your uterus during surgery because the physician decides they are no longer needed, or won't be for long, and that as long as you're having a hysterectomy, they might as well be removed too just in case they may later develop cancer. Most conservative physicians want to remove them during a hysterectomy if you are over 40.

The incidence of ovarian cancer is very low, only about 0.2 percent. On the other hand, it is a very serious cancer.

It develops silently with no symptoms and before it is detected it is often too far advanced to be easily treated.

Nevertheless, *you* are the one who must make the decision whether to take a chance on getting this very rare cancer. You must decide whether to have your ovaries removed if they are found to be perfectly healthy during a hysterectomy—at whatever age you are.

There are arguments on both sides of this question. Most specialists think that perfectly healthy ovaries should be removed during surgery if you have already passed menopause, figuring they are not much use to you anymore anyway. But even after menopause your ovaries continue to turn out *some* estrogen and androgens, perhaps for years. Many women make significant ovarian estrogen for 10 or even 15 or 20 years after menopause. Whatever amount you make, it is a protection to your arteries, your bones, your skin, and your vagina. You and your doctor must weigh these benefits against the risks.

Removing healthy ovaries *before* menopause, while they are still functioning and producing large amounts of estrogen, is yet another question. Even if you are over 40, you may have many years to go before you have menopause. To end your major estrogen supply abruptly is a serious step because of all the changes it will promptly initiate in your body.

Most younger women without ovaries receive long-term estrogen replacement to make up for it, but one's own estrogen is always the best, not only because it is made by your own body but because it is regulated according to your own individual day-to-day needs. ERT can never be as good as that.

Even if you are older, say 50 or 55, but haven't yet

reached menopause, think about it. Removing your ovaries will take away what still remains of your own hormone production, hormones that, again, could continue for years to do their job of protecting your arteries, vagina, skin, and bones though their primary function may soon be over.

If you are willing to take the chance that your ovaries will remain healthy—and those of us who don't have hysterectomies do take that chance—then you may decide to keep them. Consider the gynecologist's recommendation, get a second opinion, and remember you have an option.

IS YOUR FSH ELEVATED?

One way to help you make the decision is to have your level of circulating FSH checked out (see Chapter 12). If your FSH is elevated, you will probably have menopause within a year. Knowing this may tilt your decision toward removal. If it is not elevated, you may have years of good estrogen output left. Check with your female relatives to see when they had menopause. If, for example, your mother had hers at 58 and you are now 46, you may decide that a probable additional 12 years or so of estrogen is worth assuming the small risk of eventual ovarian problems.

No matter what you decide, however, it's a good idea to give the surgeon your written permission to remove your ovaries during the procedure if it's found they are diseased. Without that permission, you would have to have a second surgical operation a few weeks later.

12

Logistics of ERT: How, When, Where, Why

Estrogen can work wonders, producing results no other drug can accomplish anywhere near as well, but like all drugs, it must be used correctly. Here, in this section, we're going to give you the absolutely last, up-to-the-minute word on how to use it safely.

This is the most important chapter, where you will get all the information you will need about the logistics of ERT: how to take it, how you and your doctor will know if you need it, and the three alternate ways to take it—pills, patch, or vaginal cream. You'll learn the facts about the newest method of ERT, the transdermal patch, and its advantages for women who couldn't take estrogen before. You will get the latest information about dosages, precautions, possible side effects, the importance of check-ups, contraindications, and the right way to quit if you want to.

MAKING A DECISION ABOUT ESTROGEN

If your symptoms and changes aren't too severe, one of the nondrug alternatives may work well enough for you. If they don't, however, don't let your fears or your friends talk you out of estrogen therapy. Just be sure to do it *right*.

(Exception: **If you are a prime candidate for osteoporosis, don't waste valuable time trying alternatives. You must take estrogen very soon after menopause because the alternatives will not prevent the irreversible bone loss.** On the other hand, the urogenital atrophic changes, the other inevitable result of estrogen deficiency, *can* be reversed if you decide to start using estrogen later.)

———————— **Important Facts to Know Before You Begin ERT** ————

- There are women who never need ERT. Others can manage to get along without it if they want to or they must.
- There are some women who shouldn't take it, just as there are women who shouldn't take aspirin or other medications. Today because of vaginal estrogen

creams and the new transdermal patch, this group is almost exclusively limited to women who have had estrogen-dependent cancer.

• There are women who need estrogen only short-term, just long enough to get through their hot flashes or other transient vasomotor symptoms. ERT is considered short-term when it's taken anywhere from a few months to five years. With very few exceptions, every woman can safely take ERT on a short-term basis.

• There are women who need estrogen for many years or perhaps even for the rest of their lives. One of the most potent arguments for ERT long-term is to maintain the body's bone structure. There is *nothing* else that works as well to prevent or arrest osteoporosis. Nothing works as well either for persistent vaginal and urethral infections, or for vaginal changes that can turn you off sex.

• ERT is very different from oral contraceptives. The Pill *adds* hormones to a woman's already normal hormone level. The estrogen and progesterone in ERT *replace* the hormones you are no longer making for yourself and *never* give you anywhere near the amount you used to produce from your own ovaries or you would get from contraceptives.

The usual daily dose of 0.625 mg of conjugated estrogen (or the equivalent dose of other estrogen) is only about *one fifth* of the amount packed into the newest low-dose birth-control pill. It is merely a *quarter* of what we routinely gave postmenopausal women only 10 years ago.

• Occasionally, ERT causes side effects, usually quite minor and temporary, such as water retention and nausea (we'll discuss these later in this chapter). If they are uncomfortable or become a hazard, the side effects will

be promptly reversed when you stop taking the hormones.

   • Estrogen, like any other drug, should not be
taken casually. It must be prescribed individually for you
and then monitored. It must be "opposed" by progesterone if you have a uterus. And just like any other drug ever
developed, it should be taken in the smallest amount that
will accomplish its purpose.

NOT A LIFETIME COMMITMENT

   When you start ERT, you are not committed to it forever. You can stop whenever you like. You may decide
you don't require it for symptoms any longer. Or you may
decide, for whatever reason, that you don't care to take it
anymore. (If you do decide to quit, however, don't go cold
turkey. Do it according to the suggestions at the end of
the chapter.)

WHO CAN'T TAKE IT?

   Today estrogen replacement therapy is safe for virtually everyone but those who have had uterine cancer or
estrogen-dependent breast cancer. Women with these
cancers can't take estrogen because, though it is not a
carcinogenic agent and does not cause cancer, it is a
growth accelerator and can make these cancers grow if
they are already present.

(Exception: Even oncologists occasionally approve the use of ERT for ex-cancer patients who have been free of the disease for several years. The hormone is given for brief periods of time to relieve severe vaginal and/or urinary atrophic symptoms.)

You should also avoid estrogen if you have a strong family history of estrogen-dependent breast cancer.

However, if a breast tumor is found to be *non*-estrogen-dependent, which is the case in the vast majority of post-menopausal malignancies, it is not necessary to avoid hormones and, in fact, the opposite may be true. You may be treated with them instead.

Because estrogen can make large fibroids grow even larger, these benign muscle tumors may be another contraindication to long-term ERT, but not always. This is a matter of judgment and it's always possible to try ERT and see what effect it has on the fibroids (see Chapter 2). The amount of estrogen in ERT today is so small that it does not usually accelerate their growth.

NO OTHER REASONS TO AVOID ERT

You have now had a reprieve if your doctor once ruled out long-term ERT because you were already suffering from certain medical conditions such as liver impairment, gallbladder disease, renin-hypertension, or thrombophlebitis. The transdermal estrogen patch, a new development, delivers the hormone through the skin directly into the bloodstream and therefore does not affect these conditions. Vaginal estrogen cream also enters the general circulation without going through the digestive system.

This makes ERT available to you without the risk of aggravating these diseases. For more discussion, check back with Chapter 2.

ESTROGEN REPLACEMENT THERAPY: HOW IT WORKS

Estrogen and progesterone should always be taken in a physiologic way, matching the normal female body processes as closely as possible. During your reproductive years, if all is going normally, you make estrogen every single day. Then, for 13 to 14 days toward the end of the menstrual cycle, you make progesterone as well.

Most doctors prescribe ERT in the same pattern—estrogen *every* day of the month, supplemented by progesterone for a certain number of days, usually 7 to 13 days. It's quite safe, however, to take the estrogen for three weeks a month with a week off, again supplemented with progesterone every month.

PERIODS AGAIN?

Each month, when you stop taking the progesterone, you may have a brief menstrual response or period, neatly clearing out your uterus of any endometrial lining encouraged by the estrogen—just like your menstrual periods used to do. If you don't get a period in response to the progesterone, don't worry. That's even better because it means you are not getting a buildup of proliferated endometrial cells, so you don't need the period. However, you must *not* stop taking the progesterone.

Technically, what's happening is that the progesterone changes the cells of the lining from proliferative to secretory. When the progesterone is stopped after its allotted number of days, the secretions carry out all the accumulated blood and proliferated cells, leaving the endometrium clean and healthy right down to the basement membrane—just as it should be in order to be safe.

If you get periods with progesterone, they will probably last only a couple of days, and, unlike your old periods, produce only a very light or moderate flow. You may continue to have them every month for a few years; then they will stop.

Periods are not popular

The return of menstrual periods is the biggest complaint doctors hear about the new ERT. After all, most women are delighted to be rid of their periods and don't relish getting them back again after menopause. Some women, on the other hand, appreciate the new periods, associating them with youth, vigor, and good health. But, like them or not, progesterone is absolutely essential if you haven't had a hysterectomy. Frequently, women quit the progesterone because of the periods, or their doctors don't prescribe it for them because of their objections, and that is *dangerous*.

If you have a uterus, you must never stop taking progesterone unless you stop taking estrogen too. Progesterone is what makes ERT so safe today.

If you don't have a uterus, progesterone is not essential, but it's still an excellent idea to take it anyway because of its probable protection against breast cancer.

Periods are on their way out

Because most women much prefer not having the pro-gesterone-induced periods, medical researchers have been looking for a way to eliminate them safely. Though the definitive answers are not yet in, it appears that this can be accomplished. Stretching the time over which you take the progesterone to 10, 12, or 13 days a month seems to accomplish two important purposes: First, it eliminates the periods for many women. Second, it provides even better protection against overproliferation of the uterine lining. Studies made in England have shown that 10 days of progesterone a month prevents hyperplasia 98 percent of the time, while it is true 13 days may be required by a few women whose uterine linings are unusually respon-sive to estrogen.

Very recent work by Whitehead presented at the Kaiser Permanente *Tutorials in Medicine* in 1986 indicates that the pattern of bleeding in response to progesterone correlates with the amount of endometrial buildup. Women who repeatedly have a menstrual response to the progesterone within 12 hours of the last pill probably need one to two days more of the hormone than they have been taking. On the other hand, women who have no periods or who start periods 24 or more hours after stopping the proges-terone, Whitehead states, are taking adequate doses in both duration and dose.

What to expect

Your new periods, if you're going to get them, will usually start the day after you stop taking progesterone each month. The pattern should be the same every month, never varying more than 24 to 48 hours. If, for example, you take progesterone from the first to the tenth day of the month and get your menstrual response on the eleventh, you should always get it on the eleventh (give or take a day or two) every single month.

Sometimes you'll bleed one month but not the next. If you don't bleed even though you are on progesterone, great! You know your endometrium is in good shape.

If there is *any* other variation—in timing *or* flow—consider it abnormal bleeding and check it out promptly with your doctor.

––––––––––– **Bleeding: Normal or Abnormal?** –––––––––––

• When you take progesterone along with estrogen, you may have a short menstrual period just after you stop taking it each month. It will be short (two to five days), unclotted, and not very heavy. It will occur the same way every month, varying no more than one or two days, and varying only slightly in the amount of flow. This is the *only* bleeding that is allowed!

• Caution #1: If *any* bleeding occurs at *any* time other than those usual few days, it must be investigated. It is abnormal. It could be caused by polyps in the cervix or uterus. It could come from fibroids. Or it could be hyperplasia or some other problem. Whatever it is, your job is to check it out immediately.

• Caution #2: If the menstrual response to the progesterone becomes prolonged, lasting more than your usual few days, or if it contains clots, or is very heavy in flow, you must bring it promptly to the attention of your physician.

- In other words, **any bleeding that does not occur according to plan must be investigated.** There may be trouble brewing and you must look into it. Make an appointment with your doctor immediately for a complete pelvic examination, including careful scrutiny of the endometrial cells under a microscope at a reliable laboratory.

- Though the unscheduled bleeding rarely signifies a serious situation, time is important. If the doctor's office tries to put off your appointment more than two weeks, insist on an earlier one.

Periods are not forever

Even if you get them, your new periods won't continue forever. If you are on long-term therapy, they'll stop after a few years because the endometrium eventually becomes nonfunctioning and inactive. It can no longer build up any lining that must be sloughed off.

When this happens, continue taking your progesterone and don't worry. That's easy to say, but most women do get a little apprehensive when the periods disappear. They wonder what's going on, if something is wrong. But this state of affairs is perfectly normal. It simply means you now have an inactive endometrium and there's nothing to clear out each month anymore. **(Again, do *not* stop taking the progesterone as long as you take estrogen, whether or not you get periods.)**

CAN YOU GET PREGNANT?

Once you are truly menopausal, you are no longer fertile and you can't get pregnant even though you may be having menstrual responses to the progesterone. Your ovaries are not involved and you are not ovulating. Relax.

But be sure to use some kind of contraception for at least *a year* after your last real period, whether you're on ERT or not, just in case your ovaries decide to turn out one more egg. Many a woman of 45 or even 50 has been mighty surprised by this unsettling turn of events. As the doctor of some of them, I can tell you it's rarely been a happy surprise.

"PROGESTERONE MAKES ME FEEL PREMENSTRUAL"

Some women complain that progesterone makes them feel jumpy, tense, anxious, perhaps depressed, much like premenstrual tension which is also caused by a rise in the cyclical progesterone level.

Usually, these feelings are temporary, disappearing after about three months. But if they become unbearable, it's better to quit ERT altogether than to drop the progesterone. Taking estrogen without progesterone is inviting big trouble.

NO ERT BEFORE MENOPAUSE

The famous Doctor Robert Wilson, whose book *Feminine Forever* caused such a stir in the 1960s, recommended that women start taking estrogen many years before menopause, perhaps even in their 30s when their hormone level begins to taper off, and then continue for life to keep them younger and sexier by fending off the tolls of time.

Today we know that, except under special circumstances, taking hormones before menopause, your very last menstrual period, can be dangerous. In fact, it can be especially dangerous during the erratic periods of perimenopause because that's a time when you may be producing huge amounts of estrogen in response to the frantic activities of the pituitary gland to get your ovaries back in business. If you are still having periods, however irregular, that means you are still making sufficient estrogen to build up your uterine lining.

You do *not* need estrogen in addition to what you are already producing yourself. You are probably no longer ovulating and so you are not making progesterone. Without the progesterone to clean out the lining, you could develop hyperplasia. That's not cancer, but if it is allowed to continue or is stimulated to get worse, it could set the stage for it if you are predisposed.

Exception: If you have severe symptoms at this time, the physician may examine the vaginal cells under a microscope. If no cornified cells (which make up the outer layer of the vaginal lining) are found, this may mean that, even though you are still having periods, your estrogen level and your estrogen response are low. In this special instance, a brief course of ERT may be safely prescribed to stop the symptoms.

However, for other women, this may be the time to take progesterone instead, as we discussed in Chapter 3.

In any case, severe symptoms rarely make a grand entrance until after your periods are over for good.

Your estrogen level must be low and you must have had menopause *before* starting ERT. The best test for menopause, the most sensitive means of determining whether your ovarian function has diminished sufficiently and you are producing very little estrogen, is a test of your FSH serum level.

When FSH soars above 40 MIU/mL, it's all over. You know you are making very little estrogen, no progesterone at all, and your ovaries have gone into retirement. There is only one chance in a million that your FSH would be elevated for any other reason. An interesting sidelight: Once your FSH goes up, it stays up forever. Eventually your body adjusts to it.

Though there are other methods of determining whether you've really reached menopause or are about to reach it, this is the only definitive one. Measuring estrogen is very difficult and remarkably inaccurate. Cervical smears that are rated according to the amount of estrogen present can give a rough indication of your status, but are not reliable because they do not test circulating estrogen. Observation of the vagina and cervix and the presence of obvious symptoms provide clues, of course, but do not always reveal the true story.

To be sure you're safe, request an FSH test.

THE INITIAL EXAMINATION

Once you know you have reached menopause and have decided you want to start ERT to help you through

symptoms, prevent osteoporosis, ward off persistent infections, preserve your good looks, or make sex comfortable, what happens next?

These are the important preliminary steps:

——————— **Steps to Take Before ERT** ———————

1. A thorough physical examination, including
a pelvic exam and a breast exam.

2. A pap smear.

3. Complete blood tests for blood sugar, liver
function, thyroid function, cholesterol and triglyceride
levels, calcium and phosphorus levels.

4. A biopsy of your endometrium so that the
lining cells may be closely examined under a microscope.
Subsequently, your physician may decide to use the progesterone challenge test to rule out hyperplasia or cancer.
Many women and doctors prefer the challenge test because it is so simple.

5. Mammography (see page 29).

6. A complete family history, with special em-
phasis on osteoporosis and cancer.

7. Tests for existing osteoporosis if they are
deemed necessary.

FOLLOW-UP VISITS

You should have a follow-up appointment with your
doctor about three months after starting hormone therapy

to be sure you are following directions correctly. You'd be surprised how many women reverse their estrogen and progesterone doses, for example. The doctor will also check out the kind of periods you are having, make adjustments in dosage if necessary, and give you a pelvic exam to see how much your tissues are improving. Most important, you will have an opportunity to ask questions. I've found that very few women get everything straight the first time around, or at least fear they haven't. It's always best to be sure you understand the procedures and the reasoning behind them. Don't be afraid to ask every question that's lurking in your mind, no matter how trivial or embarrassing you may think it is, and make sure you get satisfying answers.

After this visit, you must return for a checkup every six months. This is important.

THREE WAYS TO TAKE ESTROGEN

Today there are three major routes for replacing the hormones you no longer make:

Oral estrogen

This is taken, as you may have guessed, by mouth in the form of tablets. Premarin—conjugated estrogen made from natural sources—is the kind most commonly prescribed all over the world today because it was introduced on the market in 1941 and in all those years it has been found to be reliable and trustworthy. It is also the estrogen on which most of the scientific testing has been done.

Today there are generic conjugated estrogens as well, plus several synthetic or semisynthetic compounds, any one of which your doctor may prescribe for you.

Oral estrogen is usually taken every day of the month, with 7 to 13 days of overlapping progesterone. Sometimes, however, physicians prefer to prescribe the estrogen for only three weeks with one week off, plus the same schedule of progesterone.

Vaginal estrogen cream

This is estrogen in cream form that is inserted into the vagina with a measured applicator. Although the hormone is absorbed into the bloodstream and affects other parts of the body, its major influence is on the tissues of the vagina and urethra where it reverses the degenerative changes caused by the lack of your natural estrogen.

For that reason, you should use this kind of estrogen only if your menopausal complaints are limited to genito-urinary problems. If you are looking for other effects from ERT, choose oral estrogen or the transdermal patch. Vaginal cream may help alleviate other symptoms, but don't count on it. If you want to prevent osteoporosis or relieve bad hot flashes, this is not the way to go.

The absorption of estrogen from the vaginal cream is very rapid at first, sending peak amounts of hormones into the bloodstream. It then slows down once the vaginal epithelium has become recornified and thickened to a younger and healthier condition.

Important: Remember you are on ERT! Most women fool themselves into thinking they aren't taking estrogen when they "only" use the cream. But they, too, are on ERT, whether they call it that or not.

That means that when you take the estrogen via vaginal estrogen cream, you will probably also need to take progesterone, at least occasionally, if you have a uterus. As we've discussed in Chapter 7, you must be checked out if you have any unplanned bleeding. Bleeding usually means you require progesterone along with your vaginal cream. And even if you don't have bleeding, it is essential to have regular endometrial biopsies or progesterone challenge tests to make sure you aren't building up too much lining from the estrogen. (This should be done even if you don't take estrogen.)

A benefit of estrogen taken vaginally is that it does not aggravate such medical conditions as liver dysfunction, hypertension, gallbladder disease, and thrombophlebitis. Like transdermal estrogen, it is not absorbed through the digestive system and so is not altered by the action of the liver.

The absorption of estrogen from vaginal cream varies incredibly, so you and your doctor will have to work out a schedule and a dose that do the job for you.

Transdermal estrogen

If you need estrogen and haven't been able to take it because it aggravated a medical condition such as gallbladder disease or hypertension, ask your doctor about this newest method of administering hormones. I'm going to take a little more time describing this method because it is so new that few women and not too many physicians even know it exists.

The first major development in estrogen replacement therapy since Premarin was developed, the transdermal therapeutic system (Estraderm) was created in a quest for a route that would avoid "the hepatic first-pass effect." This meant that the estrogen would go directly into the bloodstream without first passing through the liver circulation—thereby avoiding most of the reasons why some women couldn't take estrogen.

The transdermal therapeutic system delivers estrogen at a controlled rate into the skin and then into the general circulation, a method already long in use for other drugs such as nitroglycerin and antivertigo medications.

A small patch that looks like a round Band-Aid is applied to the skin of the abdomen and changed twice a week. Each patch contains a reservoir of hormone in a control membrane that allows a certain amount through the skin at once. This is packaged with a nonabsorbent backing and surrounding adhesive.

The patch has revolutionized ERT. When estrogen is taken into the body without passing through the digestive system and the liver, it does not cause the release of enzymes that could affect preexisting medical conditions. In addition, the estrogen remains in its purest form, estradiol, which has less tendency than other forms to cause hyperplasia.

The only apparent side effect of the patch is occasional skin irritation from the adhesive. Many women have found, however, that this reaction goes away within a few weeks of use. If not, the patch will not lose its effectiveness if it is pulled off and reapplied to a different spot whenever it begins to become bothersome. The least sensitive areas of the body, by the way, are the back and buttocks. So, if you have sensitive skin, try using the transdermal system there.

Disadvantages include the fact that the patch may not adhere properly in hot humid climates or in saunas—and may need to be reapplied. More important, a few women get insufficient estrogen absorption through the skin even though they are using a dosage equivalent to their previous oral dose, so their dosage must be increased.

Researchers at nine major medical centers across the United States—including NYU Medical Center where I directed the research—conducted a prospective double-blind controlled study comparing the transdermal system to oral estrogen. The results showed that both are equally safe and effective in reducing menopausal symptoms and reversing vaginal and urinary changes.

The final answers on its effects on calcium absorption and lipid levels are not yet in because this method hasn't been around for 40 years, but all studies so far indicate that the effects are almost identical to oral estrogen. Preliminary studies on the excretion of calcium and by-products, for example, lead us to believe it will be just as effective as oral estrogen for osteoporosis. Early lipid tests indicate that estrogen absorbed through the skin lowers the harmful LDLs as does oral estrogen but, on the other hand, does not change the levels of the beneficial HDLs.

The patch promises to be good news for women, and

―――――― **Estrogens** ――――――

TRADE NAME	AVAILABLE FORMS	MANUFACTURER
Premarin	Tablets, cream	Ayerst
Generics	Tablets	Various
Ogen	Tablets, cream	Abbott
Estrace	Tablets, cream	Mead-Johnson
Estrovis	Tablets	Reid-Provident
Dienestrol	Cream	Ortho
Estraderm	Skin patch	Ciba-Geigy

especially good news for those who need estrogen desperately but can't take it orally.

Do you need progesterone when you use the patch? Yes, you do. If you have a uterus, you must take progesterone too, just as you do with oral estrogen. This, of course, means not only remembering to change your patch twice a week but also to take a progesterone pill a day for your prescribed number of days each month.

SOME ALTERNATIVE ROUTES

Estrogen can be delivered to your body in a few other ways, but these are rarely used. They are:

Implanted subcutaneous estrogen pellets provide long-term ERT, slowly releasing the hormone for months. They eliminate the problem of remembering to take pills or patches, but the only way to stop the hormones is to remove them. Besides, if you take your estrogen this way, you must still take the progesterone by pill. The pellets have always been implanted surgically, but a new technique has been developed in Europe that places them under the skin through a catheter.

Intramuscular injection of estrogen is done only in the most unusual circumstances. Before the advent of the transdermal patch, it was given occasionally when a woman needed estrogen badly but couldn't take it by mouth.

A vaginal ring implant is in the very early stages of research and not too much is known about it yet. Its purpose is to deliver measured amounts of estradiol through the vagina.

DETERMINING ESTROGEN DOSAGES

Always take the lowest amount of any drug that will do the job assigned to it. As for estrogen, there is no need to overstimulate the endometrium with hormones so that it will build up excessively. The smallest amount of estrogen that will accomplish its various purposes is the most you should use.

What is a low dose of estrogen? In oral conjugated estrogens (Premarin), the lowest dose available is 0.3 mg. If you can get by on that, fine, but very few women can. It is such a minute amount that it's usually little more than a placebo.

In any case, in order to prevent osteoporosis you must take at least 0.625 mg of conjugated estrogen (or an equivalent amount of other estrogen), the next higher dose. This is almost always an effective amount, too, for taming hot flashes and the other assorted symptoms.

If you can't stop your flashes with 0.625 mg, however, you will still remain in the low-dose range if you require 0.9 mg, a dose that has only recently become available.

Once in a while a woman needs both oral (or patch) estrogen *plus* an occasional application of vaginal cream. One of my patients, for example, did very well on 0.625 mg of conjugated estrogen. Her flashes and other symptoms were completely relieved by this amount. But she still suffered with atrophic vaginitis which was cleared up by adding a small amount of vaginal estrogen cream every other week.

As for the transdermal patch, it is currently offered in two doses: 0.05 mg and 0.10 mg. The 0.05 mg patch is the equivalent of a daily dose of a little between 0.3 mg and 0.625 mg of estrogen. The 0.10 mg patch is approximately equivalent to between 0.9 and 1.25 mg of conjugated estrogen.

The usual dose for vaginal estrogen is one gram twice a week, though some women require a third application.

Why do doses differ?

Doses differ because every woman has her own requirements that depend, among other things, on her weight, age, and the efficiency of her estrogen receptors that make her more or less sensitive to the effects of the hormone.

In general, if you are under 40 when you have menopause, especially if it occurred because of surgery, you'll need more estrogen than if it occurred at the usual age. You may have to start with 1.25 mg of Premarin or the equivalent, then taper off later. Sometimes even more—perhaps 2.5 mg or even 5 mg, both considered high doses today—is required at least at first by women who are suffering from serious degenerative changes.

But most women do just fine with 0.625 mg or its equivalent, the lowest amount that prevents bone loss, and that's what most gynecologists will start you off with.

Once or twice a day?

Oral estrogen is almost always taken just once a day. Occasionally, though, if your symptoms are extremely severe, it's more effective to divide the dose, taking half in the morning and the other half at night. This allows a more even blood level of the hormone throughout the entire 24 hours.

Progesterone dosage

The news in progesterone dosage at this writing is that the length of time you take this second major female hormone is just as important as how much you take. According to a leader in this field, Dr. Malcolm Whitehead of King's College School of Medicine in London, whose study of thousands of women was reported in 1985, an adequate amount for most women is 5 mg of medroxyprogesterone for 10 days each month, or 10 mg for 7 days.

For other women, adjustments must be made, which is an excellent reason why you must see your doctor every six months, or whenever your bleeding seems out of the ordinary. If you bleed heavily after your progesterone each month or you develop hyperplasia, then you obviously need more because you are especially responsive to estrogen. Perhaps you require 5 or 10 mg stretched over 10 to 13 days. A 13-day schedule has been shown to eliminate the danger of hyperplasia for *every* woman tested.

For the easiest schedule to remember: Take your progesterone pills the first 10 days (or whatever number of days are prescribed for you) of every month.

"I forgot to take my pill!"

Forgetting to take your ERT pills for a couple of days isn't like forgetting birth-control pills. If you skip a day, and certainly if you skip two days, of oral contraceptives, you can assume you're not covered for that whole month and you'd better use other protection against pregnancy. But don't worry if you miss a day or two of estrogen replacement. It won't disturb the cycle and you will undoubtedly get the message to start again from a few unexpected hot flashes.

If you miss more than a couple of days, however, and you have no vasomotor symptoms at all, this may be a clue that you don't need ERT anymore (unless you are taking it long-term). Check that out with your doctor.

The same is true for the transdermal patch. Forgetting to change your patch for a couple of extra days won't do any harm, though it's a good idea not to make a habit of it.

Is ERT only now and then okay?

Doctors are constantly asked by their patients whether they can take estrogen only occasionally, say once or twice a week or only when symptoms become bothersome.

Except for the vaginal cream, it's never a good idea to take hormones only occasionally or on an irregular schedule if you haven't had a hysterectomy. This can cause incomplete endometrial buildup and the lining won't be regularly cleaned out by progesterone. The result may be bleeding or other problems. You are looking for trouble. Take your low dose every day (or twice a week if you are using the patch) and your progesterone as scheduled. Or quit the ERT. If you can get along with so little hormone, you can probably manage without any at all.

My advice: Take estrogen regularly or stop taking it altogether.

Of course, if you've had a hysterectomy, you have no

uterus to affect and so it doesn't matter so much whether you adhere to a regular schedule of estrogen.

Double dose by mistake?

If you don't have a scheduled time to take your pill, you may occasionally take two in one day by mistake—one perhaps after breakfast and another at night because you forgot about the first. It won't hurt you if you don't make a habit of it and end up overdosing yourself.

The best time for the pill is usually just before bed. If you always take it when you brush your teeth at night, you'll remember, and you'll know you haven't taken one earlier that day.

If you use the transdermal patch, you'll never put on a second one; however, you might forget to change it. So if you use the transdermal patch that is changed twice a week, make yourself a schedule—say, Monday and Thursday just before bed—and post it over your bathroom sink to remind you. Again, the world won't end if you forget. If you start getting symptoms again, you'll remember!

CAN ORAL CONTRACEPTIVES BE USED FOR ERT?

Definitely not. They contain much much more estrogen than you need or should have, as well as much more progesterone. They can cause clotting problems in older women, which normal ERT doses do not, and other complications too. Birth-control pills should not be taken for any reason after the age of 35.

Oral contraceptives won't prevent menopause—a myth that has become widely circulated—but they will cause you to continue having periods because of the estrogen/progesterone combination. So you won't know if you have had menopause or not! Eventually, probably around the age of 60, the endometrium will become inactive and the periods will stop. Taking The Pill this long is an exceedingly dangerous practice.

Sometimes when you stop taking The Pill, your own estrogen production doesn't get going again immediately. This could happen because of a lag from the years when there was no need to make your own—or it could be you've had early menopause. If you stop taking it at an age when you wouldn't expect to be menopausal, and your periods don't begin again within two months, go to a gynecologist or endocrinologist and have some tests made. You should know your status. If you haven't reached menopause, you may need help to encourage your ovaries to get to work again.

If your ovaries don't get going quickly, it's quite possible you'll have hot flashes, sweats, or other menopausal symptoms—whether or not you're truly in menopause. In fact, you can expect them because, for this moment, you *are* menopausal because of the sudden drop in estrogen.

If you *have* had menopause (even though it has been disguised by the effects of The Pill) when you quit the oral contraceptives, you will probably have the most severe symptoms. It's very similar to the response experienced after a surgical menopause—you are suffering from both the abrupt withdrawal of estrogen and the sudden rush of FSH. If this happens, go to your gynecologist and get help.

IS IT EVER TOO LATE FOR ERT?

If you need it, it's never too late. At any age, estrogen will prevent your bones from becoming thinner than they already are, though it can't restore the bone you have lost. It will rejuvenate your vaginal and urinary tissues, reconditioning your sex life and resistance to persistent infections. I've had many patients come to me in their 70s and 80s, and sometimes 90s, and even then, ERT can work wonders.

If you wait many years before seeking help, however, you may require a high dose of estrogen at first and the beneficial results may take longer to occur. Eventually the hormones will work, though perhaps not as well as they would have if you had moved more quickly. Sometimes long years of estrogen deficiency cause such extensive degeneration of the vaginal and urinary tissues that they can never be completely restored, but in most instances you'd be amazed by what ERT can do.

REMEMBER YOUR CHECKUPS

When you are on ERT, you must have a checkup every six months. In fact, I strongly advise this schedule whether or not you take estrogen.

At each visit, the routine should include complete pelvic and breast examinations, Pap smear, and blood tests.

If there's any indication of hyperplasia or any other uterine problem, an aspiration biopsy is essential for examination of the endometrial cells. A Pap smear is *not* sufficient because it is designed only for cervical examination and will not pick up abnormal tissue in the uterus.

When you are on long-term oral estrogen, the doctor should check for possible aggravation of previous conditions: again, hypertension, liver function, gallbladder function, or clotting problems.

THE POSSIBLE SIDE EFFECTS OF ERT

Estrogen replacement sometimes causes side effects. Usually these are minor and transient, but occasionally they are serious enough or uncomfortable enough to warrant abandoning the therapy. They are all completely reversible when treatment is stopped.

Fluid retention

This is the most common side effect and occurs in about half the women on ERT. Most of the time it only lasts for a few weeks and then vanishes. If it doesn't go away, you can probably get relief by cutting down on salt or taking an occasional diuretic. Try taking 100 to 500 mg a day of vitamin B6, a natural diuretic. Fluid retention isn't a serious complication, but about 2 out of every 100 women consider it reason enough to quit the hormones.

Tender breasts

You may find your breasts become full and tender soon after you start estrogen replacement, just as they did before your periods. This is almost always temporary and nothing to worry about. The discomfort is a result of fluid retention and stimulated mammary glands. It usually goes away within a few weeks, or at least becomes tolerable. But sometimes it doesn't and can be a reason to stop ERT or to try the lowest possible dose. For some women, taking progesterone for more days will take care of the problem.

Weight gain

About a quarter of the women who take estrogen report a gain of two or even a few more pounds when they first start the therapy. It's probably a result of the water retention and of estrogen's tendency to encourage fat tissue, just as the male hormones encourage muscle tissue.

Confusing the issue is the fact that women tend to gain weight anyway after menopause and that their bodies are busy redistributing their fat. But usually women on ERT will gain in the hips and breasts and lose in their waists and backs—just the opposite of estrogen-deficient women.

Nausea

A few women will feel slightly nauseated when they first start taking oral estrogen, but this is usually a transient situation. If this happens to you, try taking the pill just before you go to bed so the feeling will arrive while you're sleeping. In a couple of weeks, the problem will undoubtedly be gone. If not, try the transdermal patch which sends estrogen through the skin rather than the stomach, eliminating the possibility of nausea.

Vaginal discharge

Taking hormones can produce a supersupply of vaginal lubrication. This has no medical consequence but it certainly can be a nuisance. Douching with a mild solution of vinegar may help.

Headaches

Once in a great while, women complain that estrogen supplements give them headaches, especially if they tend to get migraines. The most likely explanation is increased fluid retention in the brain or change in vascular reactivity. If the headaches don't go away on the lowest dose of estrogen, you may have to forgo the treatment.

Estrogen allergy

It's possible to be allergic to almost anything, and once in a while a woman is allergic to estrogen supplements. They can cause rashes, swollen tongue, itching—all the typical allergic responses. Sometimes a different brand or method of estrogen replacement will solve the problem, but sometimes the only answer is to quit.

TIME TO QUIT?

If you're taking ERT only long enough to live through your symptoms comfortably, you'll probably need it for only about two years. But you won't know whether it's time to stop until you try it. Taper off gradually, as explained below, and see if the symptoms return. If they do, you may want to continue the estrogen (and progesterone, of course) for a while longer until you can stop without major discomfort.

HOW TO QUIT ERT

Never quit hormones abruptly. Don't go cold turkey or you may promptly start having severe symptoms because of the rebound response from the pituitary gland. This can happen no matter how long you've been on ERT or whether you were still having symptoms before you began it. The pituitary is stimulated by the sudden loss of estrogen and, as a result, produces massive amounts of FSH which, in turn, stimulates the hypothalamus and makes your temperature-regulating mechanism go haywire.

Always go off ERT very gradually. Cut back to every other day and hold it there for a month. Then take the pills only twice a week for a month; then once a week for a few weeks.

During this gradual withdrawal, continue to take your usual amount of progesterone each month.

If you no longer need estrogen for symptoms, you probably won't get them now. If you do, you'll know it soon enough and you can always go back to ERT.

LONG-TERM THERAPY

If you are taking long-term estrogen therapy, there's no need to stop the hormones for "a rest" no matter how many years pass by, unless you develop side effects or hyperplasia. It is quite safe to take it for a lifetime to prevent brittle bones and the degeneration of vaginal and urinary tissues—if you remember the important guidelines: low doses, progesterone if you haven't had a hysterectomy, a checkup every six months or whenever you have bleeding that's not according to plan.

YOU'RE NOT IN THIS ALONE

Don't ever think you can safely be your own doctor when you are taking estrogen replacement therapy—or any other drug, for that matter. To begin with, you need a doctor to write the prescriptions which are usually not automatically renewable. More important, you need a competent and knowledgeable physician for your regular checkups.

Remember, this is your one and only body. If you want it to last you a lifetime in good condition, give it the best of care!

13

Doctor,
Is This
Normal?

It is an excellent idea to know your body well enough to notice whether anything is going on that's different or perhaps abnormal. During perimenopause and for a few years after menopause, that's sometimes hard to do because your body is changing and you may not know what's normal and what isn't. Your body does feel different very often and new things are happening.

That's why the more information you have about menopause, the better. This is a time when many women become very concerned about their health, not only because of the physical changes but because, for them, menstruation has always been the symbol of feminine health. Certainly every woman finds erratic periods and strange sensations to be unsettling.

For many reasons, it is important to have regular checkups with a competent and knowledgeable doctor about every six months, and to report to that doctor whenever you have any indication that something might be wrong. Keep in mind that it's always best to be safe. Don't worry about being a nuisance.

HEAVY PERIODS: GO TO YOUR DOCTOR

Women in perimenopause often have very copious menstrual periods sometimes accompanied by clots, almost like minor hemorrhages.

Is this normal? Yes. Should it be ignored? No. Although the heavy flow is almost surely due to hormonal changes, there is always a small possibility something is wrong. This is the most common time for hyperproliferation to occur, in other words, for the endometrium to build up abnormally into hyperplasia, which should not be allowed to continue.

This can be easily investigated by your physician. With two or three months of treatment with progesterone, taken for one week of each month, the uterine lining can almost always be stimulated to shed any excessive buildup and return to normal periods. If this happens, you will know the heavy periods can be explained by lack of ovulation and progesterone.

If the periods don't become normal, however, then the bleeding should be considered abnormal and further investigation is essential.

BLEEDING AT UNSCHEDULED TIMES: GO TO YOUR DOCTOR

Whenever you have bleeding or spotting at times other than during your periods or the miniperiods produced by estrogen/progesterone therapy, consider it abnormal and report it to your doctor. Be sure to have an examination promptly.

The bleeding may be caused by hyperplasia, polyps (small benign growths), fibroids, or some other problem. Once in a great while, a woman who is not taking ERT will have spotting because of atrophic vaginitis. The lining of the vagina becomes so raw, thin, and irritable that it bleeds easily, especially after intercourse.

After your periods have stopped for about six months, consider any new bleeding to be reason for an examination even though it is quite possible—and normal—for your periods to reappear again after such a long time. Check with your doctor, too, if you have periods at less than three-week intervals.

FIBROIDS EXPLAINED

Fibroids are nonmalignant tumors composed mostly of muscle and fibrous connective tissue. You can get them at any age but they are most usual after 35 or 40, and more than 40 percent of all women over 50 have them. Usually they appear in clusters, remain small, and are not a source of trouble.

Fibroids are the most common cause of abnormal bleeding, usually in extraheavy periods. They are seldom painful and they are not inherently dangerous. If they don't cause problems, there is no need to do anything about them. Sometimes, however, they grow so large that they cause bleeding or apply pressure on the bladder, ureter, or rectum. If that happens, a hysterectomy may be your only recourse.

The Doctor's Examination

If there is any question that all is not well, an exploration and examination of the cervix and uterus must be made by your doctor. And it should be followed up at least every six months.

These are the usual procedures for determining the status of your endometrium:

1. *Pap smear.* A few cells from the lower end of the cervix are scraped off with a wooden spatula and examined under a microscope. A Pap smear may give you a sense of security when the results of the test are negative, but it is a false sense of security because the smear tests only the cells of the cervix. It is *not* a reliable test for endometrial cancer.

2. *Progesterone challenge test.* As we explained above, this is an excellent way to test the endometrium. The doctor will prescribe progesterone, probably 10 mg a day for seven days. If the progesterone regulates perimen-

opausal periods, making them become regular and normal in flow and timing, this is an excellent indication that nothing abnormal is going on.

After menopause, the progesterone challenge test is frequently used instead of an endometrial biopsy as a check for hyperplasia. If the progesterone doesn't produce any bleeding after it's stopped, it's most unlikely that hyperplasia is present. If you do bleed and further tests show you have hyperplasia, this condition can almost invariably be reversed with two or three months of progesterone treatment.

3. *Endometrial biopsy.* An office procedure, the biopsy is usually done today with suction instruments which do not dilate the cervix and therefore are not very uncomfortable. Because this method gets close to 98 percent accuracy, it eliminates the need for many D&Cs. A small tube is inserted through the cervix into the uterus, then suction is used to trap cells for examination. Some physicians still remove samples of the uterine lining with a cutting rather than a suction instrument.

4. *D&C (dilation and curettage).* This is a minor medical procedure usually performed in the hospital with general anesthesia. The cervix is dilated and expanded with instruments and the uterine lining is scraped and removed, and small pieces of tissue are examined under a microscope by a pathologist.

A D&C is never done routinely, but only to investigate abnormal bleeding or an enlargement of the uterus. Occasionally it is also performed when polyps have been found in the cervix and the doctor wants to know if there are more in the uterus.

FINDING THE RIGHT DOCTOR

Most women spend more time shopping for a new car or buying a coat than they do for a doctor. But choosing the right doctor is far more important than almost any other decision you'll ever need to make. There may come a critical moment when your future is in that person's hands, and that's no time to discover you haven't made the best choice. If you are typical of most women, you see a doctor only when you have a problem and, at that point, you may be strangers to one another. You can't be sure you're getting the best treatment if you haven't established a relationship or had a chance to check this person out.

Most women find doctors through the recommendations of friends or relatives. If your friends or relatives are the kind of people who investigate their choices thoroughly, fine. But usually *they* found the doctor through their next-door neighbor's second cousin who heard about this physician through her hairdresser. It's safer not to rely solely on such references. This is an important decision.

Shop around for a doctor, just as you would for a car. It's usually best to choose a doctor recommended by another doctor you trust. Ask questions, get opinions from patients, poll your friends, check credentials and affiliations in such reference books as the *Directory of Medical Specialists,* found in most public libraries. If you're really stumped, call or write the chief of medicine at the best hospital in your area and ask for a recommendation. You may also be able to investigate physicians through public-interest groups in your community. Consumer organizations in many states have prepared consumers' guides to doctors.

Once you've got a recommendation of a doctor, your decision should still be up in the air. This doctor may be excellent at his or her trade but poor in human relations. You should find someone who gives you what you need. Some women want to be told what to do; others want to share in the decision-making. The relationship must be a comfortable one that satisfies you intellectually and emotionally.

You must be able to talk to your doctor, to confide and discuss even the most delicate subjects. You must feel that you are not being rushed out of the office before you've asked all the questions you want to ask—and have received satisfying answers. You need a good listener who won't be affronted by naive questions or strong opinions. The doctor may have gone through menopause before with hundreds of patients, but you haven't!

Your doctor should never treat you so authoritatively or casually that you're not asked for your feelings about the problem and the treatment. Everything should be explained and discussed. This is especially true at menopause because this doctor may have views about it that don't match yours.

After you've chosen a doctor, remember you are not married to this person and you don't need a divorce if the match doesn't work out. If you don't think you are getting the best care or if your personalities don't mesh, don't go back. Find someone who suits you better.

DO YOU NEED A GYNECOLOGIST?

Every woman, especially after 40, should have a complete pelvic examination at least once a year and every six months if she is on medication such as hormone replacement. Many generalists and internists consider the female reproductive system part of their bailiwick and routinely do all their own pelvic exams. If they run into a question or a problem they can't handle, they will (or should) send you to a gynecologist who is a specialist in the female reproductive processes.

This is perfectly legitimate, to my mind, though I believe that specialists are always best when anything out of the ordinary is taking place in your body. A gynecologist sees many more cases of vaginal infections, delivers more babies, has dealt with more women at menopause, is more knowledgeable about estrogen replacement therapy, and is more likely to have kept up with the most recent developments in the field than an internist.

In most cases, it would be ideal for you to have a general doctor *and* a gynecologist. You should see the internist or family doctor once a year for a complete checkup and the specialist at least once a year for a pelvic examination, whether or not you think you have a problem.

And let's not forget the reproductive endocrinologists, like myself, who specialize in women's glands and the hormones they secrete. The endocrinologist has always trained first as an internist or gynecologist before going on to this more sophisticated field.

You will never see an endocrinologist as a matter of routine, but only when there is a question of hormonal dysfunction. If you are having great difficulties, if there are questions about whether or not you should have hormone therapy, if there are doubts about how the therapy should be carried out, then the internist or gynecologist may recommend a consultation with an endocrinologist.

If your doctor does not recommend a consultation, but you have strong doubts about how your case is being handled or think you need the opinion of a hormone specialist, suggest it yourself or arrange to see a specialist on your own.

14

Fight Back!
It's Your Own
Body!

IN THIS BOOK, we've tried to answer every question you have ever wanted to ask about menopause and estrogen, to give you the facts and the fictions, the history and the science, the trade-offs and the alternatives, so you can decide for yourself what's going on inside of you and what you want to do about it. You're probably going to live another 30, 40, or even 50 years beyond menopause, and what you choose to do can make a remarkable difference in the quality of those years.

MARTYRS AND STOICS ARE OUT OF STYLE

Menopause isn't a disease and so it needn't be cured. It is simply a natural and normal phase of life. But when that becomes a difficult phase, my advice is to look for help. I'm sure you've already found out that I believe martyrs and stoics are out of style.

I'll tell you again what I tell my patients: Fight back! Refuse to suffer needlessly. Don't accept major discomforts or disabilities when you don't have to. Take charge of your own body whenever you can. And make your own decisions—with the help, of course, of a competent and knowledgeable physician.

Deal with menopausal problems in the same way you'd deal with any other physical problem. Learn everything you can about your situation. Decide if you need help and make sure you get it if you do. First, try the nonmedical alternatives.

Prepare as much as you can, too, for menopause by eating well, following good living habits, taking care of your body, staying in condition, and maintaining emotional equilibrium. I'm sure it's true that women who build their physical and mental health through healthy living are probably best prepared for an easy passage through this time of change.

But sometimes, no matter how prepared you are, how healthy, how well-conditioned, how sane and occupied and fulfilled you've been, how many vitamins, minerals, quarts of cranberry juice, and containers of yogurt you consume, you are still going to have disabling hot flashes, palpitations, tingling fingers, or sleepless nights. If you're susceptible, you're still going to develop brittle bones that break for no good reason or end up with a vagina that's physically incapable of sexual intercourse.

Sometimes more help is required—and you have a right to have it.

ERT WITHOUT FEAR

I certainly don't recommend estrogen replacement therapy for everyone because not every woman needs it or wants it. But it is now considered a safe and effective alternative for those who do. It won't turn the clock back and it won't keep you young forever, but on the other hand, it can work wonders when you desperately need its services.

YOU'VE GOT A CHOICE

Today you have a real choice about whether you're going to take estrogen to replace the hormones you no longer make for yourself, because now we know that, taken correctly, estrogen won't hurt you. It won't cause cancer or any other dire disease and, in fact, it can protect you against it. You can take the hormone systemically with pills or patches, or topically with vaginal cream. You can take it only as long as it helps you and stop taking it whenever you want to—or you can take it for the rest of your days without danger if you follow the rules.

That means it's really up to you. It's your choice. Isn't it wonderful that we've come so far?

Bibliography

Avioli, L. V. "Postmenopausal Osteoporosis: Prevention Versus Cure." *Federal Proceedings* 40 (1981): 2418.

Aylward, M. "Estrogens, Plasma Tryptophan Levels in Perimenopausal Patients." Chap. 12 in S. Campbell, ed., *The Management of the Menopause and Postmenopausal Years.* London: University Park Press, 1975, pp. 135–47.

Bush, T. L., L. D. Cowen, E. Barrett-Connor, et al. "Estrogen Use and All-Cause Mortality: Preliminary Results from the Lipid Research Clinics Program Follow-up Study." *Journal of the American Medical Association* 249 (1983): 903–6.

Campbell, S. "Double Blind Psychometric Studies on the Effects of a Natural Estrogen on Postmenopausal Women." Chap. 13 in S. Campbell, ed., *The Management of the Menopause and Postmenopausal Years.* London: University Park Press, 1975.

Campbell, S., and M. Whitehead. "Oestrogen Therapy and the Menopausal Syndrome." *Clinical Obstetrics and Gynaecology* 4 (1977): 31–47.

Casper, R. F., S. S. C. Yen, and M. M. Wilkes. "Menopausal Flushes: Neuroendocrine Link with Pulsatile LH Release." *Science* 205 (1980): 823–25.

Danielle, H. W. "Osteoporosis of the Slender Smoker: Vertebral Compression Fractures and Loss of Metacarpal Cortex in Relation to Postmenopausal Cigarette Smoking and Lack of Obesity." *Archives of Internal Medicine* 136 (1976): 298.

Danielle, H. W. "Postmenopausal Tooth Loss." *Archives of Internal Medicine* 143 (1983): 1678.

Eskin, B. A. "Aging and the Menopause." In B. A. Eskin, ed., *The Menopause, Comprehensive Management*. New York: Masson, 1980, pp. 73–92.

Gambrell, Jr., R. D. "Estrogens, Progestogens, and Endometrial Cancer." *Journal of Reproductive Medicine* 18 (1977): 301–6.

Gambrell, Jr., R. D., R. C. Maier, and B. T. Sanders. "Decreased Incidence of Breast Cancer in Postmenopausal Estrogen-Progestogen Users." *Obstetrics and Gynecology* 62 (1983): 435.

Gambrell, Jr., R. D., F. M. Massey, and T. A. Castaneda. "Reduced Incidence of Endometrial Cancer Among Postmenopausal Women Treated with Progestogens." *Journal of the American Geriatric Society* 27 (1979): 389–94.

Gambrell, Jr., R. D., C. A. Bagnell, and R. B. Greenblatt. "Role of Estrogens and Progesterone in the Etiology and Prevention of Endometrial Cancer: A Review." *American Journal of Obstetrics and Gynecology* 146 (1983): 696.

Gambrell, Jr., R. D., F. M. Massey, and T. A. Castaneda. "Use of the Progestogen Challenge Test to Reduce the Risk of Endometrial Cancer." *Obstetrics and Gynecology* 55 (1980): 732–38.

Greenblatt, R. C. Nezhat, and A. Karpas. "The Menopausal Syndrome: Hormone Replacement Therapy." In B. A. Eskin, ed., *The Menopause: Comprehensive Management*. New York: Masson, 1980, pp. 151–72.

Hammond, C. B., F. R. Jelousick, and K. L. Lee. "Effects of

Long-term Estrogen Replacement Therapy." II. "Neoplasia." *American Journal of Obstetrics and Gynecology* 133 (1979): 537.

Hammond, C. B., and W. S. Maxson. "Current Status of Estrogen Therapy for the Menopause." *Fertility and Sterility* 37 (1982): 5–25.

Henderson, B. E., et al. "Menopausal Estrogen Therapy and Hip Fractures." *Annals of Internal Medicine* 95 (1981): 28.

Lindsay, R., D. M. Hart, J. M. Ahkem, et al. "Long-term Prevention of Postmenopausal Osteoporosis by Oestrogen." *Lancet* 2 (1976): 1038.

Lindsay, R., D. M. Hart, and D. M. Clark. "The Minimum Effective Dose of Estrogen for Prevention of Postmenopausal Bone Loss." *Obstetrics and Gynecology* 63 (1984): 759–63.

McKinlay, S., N. Bifano, and J. McKinlay. "Smoking and Age at Menopause in Women." *Annals of Internal Medicine* 103 (1985): 350.

Meldrum, D. R., I. V. Tataryn, A. M. Frumar, et al. "Gonadotropins, Estrogens, and Adrenal Steroids During Menopausal Hot Flash." *Journal of Clinical Endocrinology and Metabolism* 50 (1980): 585–89.

Nachtigall, L., R. H. Nachtigall, R. D. Nachtigall, et al. "Estrogens and Endometrial Carcinoma: Correspondence." *New England Journal of Medicine* 294 (1976): 848.

Nachtigall, L., R. H. Nachtigall, R. D. Nachtigall, et al. "Estrogen Therapy I: A 10-Year Prospective Study in the Relationship to Osteoporosis." *Obstetrics and Gynecology* 53 (1979): 277–80.

Regestein, Q. R., I. Schiff, D. Tulchinsky, et al. "Relationships Among Estrogen-Induced Psychophysiological Changes in Hypogonadal Women." *Psychosomatic Medicine* 43 (1981): 147–55.

Schiff, I., D. Tulchinsky, and K. Ryan. "Vaginal Absorption

of Estrone and 17-β-estradiol." *Fertility and Sterility* 28 (1977): 1063–66.

Schiff, I., Q. Regestein, and J. Schinfeld, et al. "Interactions of Oestrogens and Hours of Sleep on Cortisol, FSH, LH, Prolactin in Hypogonadal Women." *Maturitas* 2 (1980): 179–83.

Siiteri, P. K., B. E. Swartz, and P. C. MacDonald. "Estrogen Receptors and the Estrone Hypothesis in Relation to Endometrial and Breast Cancer." *Gynecological Oncology* 2 (1974): 228–38.

Smith, P. "Postmenopausal Urinary Symptoms and Hormonal Replacement Therapy." *British Medical Journal* 2 (1976): 941.

Stampfer, M. J., W. C. Willett, G. A. Colditz, et al. "A Prospective Study of Postmenopausal Estrogen Therapy and Coronary Heart Disease." *New England Journal of Medicine* 313 (1985): 1044.

Tataryn, I. V., D. R. Meldrum, K. H. Lu, et al. "LH, FSH, and Skin Temperature During the Menopausal Hot Flash." *Journal of Clinical Endocrinology and Metabolism* 49 (1979): 152–54.

Thom, M. H., P. J. White, R. M. Williams, et al. "Prevention and Treatment of Endometrial Disease in Climacteric Women Receiving Oestrogen Therapy." *Lancet* 1 (1979): 455–57.

Vandenbroucke, J., J. C. M. Whitteman, H. A. Malkenburg, et al. "Noncontraceptive Hormones and Rheumatoid Arthritis in Perimenopausal and Postmenopausal Women." *Journal of the American Medical Association* 255 (1986): 1299.

Whitehead, M. I., I. McQueen, J. Minardi, et al. "Clinical Considerations in the Management of the Menopause: The Endometrium." *Postgraduate Medical Journal* 54 (Suppl. 2) (1978): 69–73.

INDEX